PROGRESSIVE
EXERCISE THERAPY

PROGRESSIVE EXERCISE THERAPY

IN REHABILITATION
AND PHYSICAL EDUCATION

BY

JOHN H. C. COLSON, F.C.S.P., F.S.R.G., M.B.A.O.T.

*Former Director of Rehabilitation, Pinderfields General Hospital,
and sometime Principal, School of Remedial Gymnastics and
Recreational Therapy*

WITH A FOREWORD BY

PROFESSOR J. M. P. CLARK, M.B.E., M.B., Ch.B., F.R.C.S.

THIRD EDITION

BRISTOL
JOHN WRIGHT & SONS LTD.
1975

First Edition, 1958
Second Edition, 1969
Third Edition, 1975

ISBN 0 7236 0354 5

PRINTED IN GREAT BRITAIN BY JOHN WRIGHT & SONS LTD.
AT THE STONEBRIDGE PRESS, BRISTOL BS4 5NU

The Wise, for Cure, on Exercise depend.—DRYDEN.

PREFACE

THE importance of progression in specific exercise therapy is well recognized, but in practice seldom receives the attention it deserves. As a result treatment is either unnecessarily prolonged or fails to achieve its purpose.

The third edition of this book provides (as before) a comprehensive collection of free exercises for all parts of the body, graded and progressed in strength and mobility from the simplest to the most strenuous movement. The exercise 'vocabulary' is supplemented by a section on methods of progression, together with an evaluation of the various types of resisted exercises and their technique of progression.

To illustrate the way in which the vocabulary may be used when planning exercise programmes, a section has been devoted to the exercise treatment of various general surgical and orthopædic conditions. The range of conditions included has been limited to keep this section of the book within reasonable bounds.

The final part of the book outlines the modern approach to general exercise therapy by the use of circuit training and exercises to music, and includes specimen circuits and warming-up programmes.

A new section has been included on the use of music and movement and game-form activities in the treatment of the mentally handicapped and the mentally ill. I believe this will be of help to remedial and caring staff working in subnormality and psychiatric hospitals. In the past there has been a dearth of information not only about the scope of recreational therapy, but (what is equally important) the practical ways and means of getting it across to patients.

My sincere thanks are due to John M. P. Clark, Emeritus Professor of Orthopædic Surgery, University of Leeds, for his Foreword and for his constant encouragement and advice. I should also like to thank Mr. Robert Bremner, F.R.C.S., and Mr. C. Denley Clark, F.R.C.S., for help with certain clinical aspects of the book.

PREFACE

My grateful thanks are due as well to Mr. W. J. Armour, M.C.S.P., M.S.R.G., Principal of the College of Remedial Gymnastics and Recreational Therapy, for his advice and criticism. I must also thank the many physiotherapists and remedial gymnasts who assisted me in testing and grading the exercises arranged in Part 2 of the book—in particular, Mr. Frank Collison, M.S.R.G., who gave freely of his scanty leisure time.

Thanks are also due to Mr. R. Wells, who gave me valuable assistance when I was planning the section on mental illness; Mr. R. Gordon and Mr. W. McNeil, both remedial gymnasts with a wide experience of recreational therapy in the treatment of the mentally handicapped; the publishers who have so generously allowed me to quote from various textbooks; and the artist, Mr. S. Francis, whose diagrams help to explain the text so well. Finally, I should like to thank my publishers, Messrs. John Wright & Sons, Ltd., for their unfailing co-operation and courtesy.

JOHN C. H. COLSON

CONTENTS

PART IV: GENERAL EXERCISE THERAPY

FOREWORD

THE call for a third edition of this excellent book is testimony to the need which it has already supplied and is likely to continue to supply in the future. Since the second edition the author has had the opportunity to extend his field of operation into the realms of mental handicap and psychiatric illness with a success to be expected from the soundness of the basic principles he has for so long inculcated. Mr. Colson, in spreading his influence to new endeavours and to the remedial world at large, has indeed emulated the achievement so succinctly phrased in Alexander Pope's couplet:

> By nature honest, by experience wise,
> Healthy by temperance, and by exercise.

JOHN M. P. CLARK

PART I

SPECIFIC EXERCISE THERAPY

CHAPTER I

GENERAL CONSIDERATIONS

SPECIFIC or local exercises consist of active movements which are designed to restore function. They are used to develop a particular muscle group, mobilize a particular joint, or re-educate neuromuscular co-ordination, and are of the greatest value in the treatment of injuries and disorders of the locomotor system where certain muscle groups and joints are affected and the rest are comparatively normal, e.g., in fractures and other bone and joint injuries, thoracic diseases, and post-operative abdominal conditions.

Specific exercises are not sufficient in themselves to bring about perfect functional recovery, however, for muscle and joints were never intended by nature to act as individualists. For the best results specific exercises must be combined with general exercises, so as to co-ordinate the movements of the affected part with the rest of the locomotor system. It is also frequently necessary to combine treatment by exercises with occupational therapy, passive therapy, and recreational therapy: games, swimming, walking, and cycling.

TYPES OF SPECIFIC EXERCISES

Specific exercises consist of Free movements, Resisted movements, and Assisted movements.

Assisted movements are performed by the patient with the assistance of the therapist or some outside force (i.e., sling suspension units or cord-and-pulley circuits) and are not considered in this book.

Free Exercises

Free exercises are performed by the patient without external assistance or resistance (beyond that exerted by gravity), although in some instances they are controlled by apparatus. They consist of simple, everyday anatomical movements and gymnastic exercises drawn from the main systems of physical education in use today.

Free movements are not confined to any one phase of recovery, although the gymnastic type of movement is reserved more especially for the intermediate and final phases. In general, they are employed more often than any other form of remedial exercises, because they make the patient rely on his own efforts, are particularly suitable for group and class work, and do not require specialized equipment beyond the normal type of gymnasium apparatus.

Resisted Exercises

Resisted exercises are those in which the prime mover muscles work against the resistance of some outside force. Resistance may be given by (a) apparatus (weights, weight-and-pulley circuits, springs, or frictional apparatus), (b) the patient, and (c) the therapist.

In applying resistance to muscles three rules must be observed:

1. The resistance should be given *smoothly* from the beginning to the end of the movement.

2. It should diminish gradually from the beginning to the end of the movement, so as to conform to the physiological principle that muscles are capable of exerting their greatest force when they are fully extended, and that as they shorten their force diminishes.

3. A brief period of complete relaxation should follow each muscular effort.

Weight-and-pulley Resistance

The weight-and-pulley circuit can be easily adapted to conform to these rules. The application of gradually decreasing resistance is based on the principle that the leverage of resistance decreases as the line of application of the resistance approaches the fulcrum. In other words, the maximum effort of a given resistance on muscles is obtained when it is arranged at right-angles to the long axis of the moving limb, while the nearer the force is applied in line with the long axis of the limb the less is the resistance offered to the muscles.

Figs. 1 and 2 indicate the principle of diminishing resistance as applied to the extensor muscles of the knee. *Fig.* 2 shows how

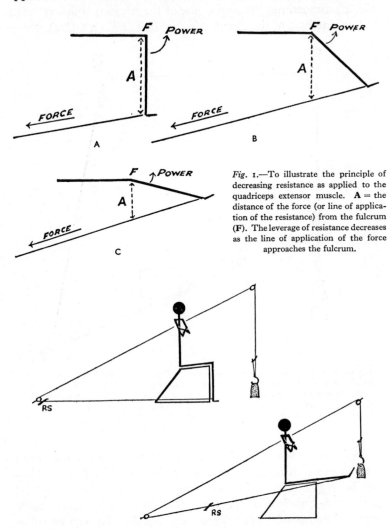

Fig. 1.—To illustrate the principle of decreasing resistance as applied to the quadriceps extensor muscle. **A** = the distance of the force (or line of application of the resistance) from the fulcrum (**F**). The leverage of resistance decreases as the line of application of the force approaches the fulcrum.

Fig. 2.—Diagrammatic representation of a simple method of applying weight-and-pulley resistance to the quadriceps extensor muscle. RS represents the relaxation stop, which frees the muscle from resistance 'pull' in the resting position.

relaxation for the working muscles is obtained in the starting and
finishing positions by a simple relaxation stop incorporated into
the circuit. The stop consists of a rectangular-shaped piece of
wood or metal provided with three holes to take the cord. (*See
Fig.* 4.) Sometimes the stop is one of the wooden 'runners' used
to link one part of the circuit with another (*Figs.* 3 and 4).

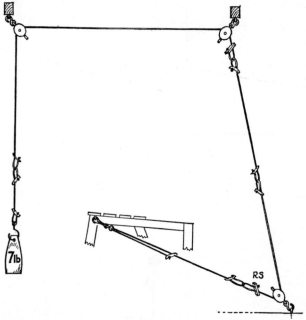

Fig. 3.—Plan of an alternative type of weight-and-pulley circuit for the quadriceps extensor
muscle. It is used when the height of the pulley-room or gymnasium is limited and less than
14 ft. Note that the relaxation stop (RS) consists of one of the ordinary wooden 'runners'
used on the circuit cord to adjust its length (cf. with *Fig.* 4). The circuit is fastened to a
leather strap (worn on the patient's foot and ankle) by a strong spring-hook and swivel of
the dog-lead variety.

Equipment.—Weight-and-pulley circuits can be constructed
without much difficulty or expense, as indicated by *Fig.* 4. They
can be rigged up in the gymnasium or (preferably) a special
pulley-room; their disadvantage is that they require considerable
space. Alternatively, specialized weight-and-pulley equipment is
available which allows a wide range of resisted movements: the
Armour Exerciser, for example, which has the advantage of being
portable.

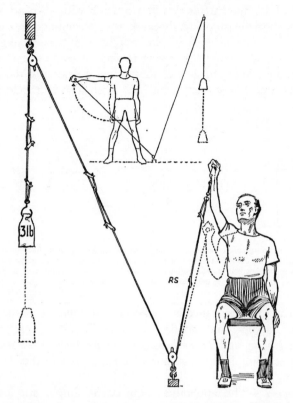

Fig. 4.—Details of a weight-and-pulley circuit used to give resistance to the elevator muscles of the arm: elevation through abduction. RS indicates a three-holed relaxation stop. *Inset*: The circuit used to strengthen the abductor muscles of the shoulder-joint. The handle of the circuit is of the wood-and-metal type supplied with spring-resistance units. It is fastened to the circuit by a strong spring-hook and swivel.

WEIGHT RESISTANCE

Resistance by weights is most efficient and useful in practice, but it has the disadvantage that when it is applied to the muscle groups of the limbs in the standing and sitting positions, it increases from the beginning to the end of all movements made within an arc of 90° from the vertical plane, because the perpendicular distance between the line of pull of the weight and the moving joint increases (*Fig.* 5).

When weight resistance is applied to the muscles of the limbs in the lying position, however, it decreases from the beginning to

the end of all movements which are made within an arc of 90°
from the horizontal plane, because the perpendicular distance
between the line of pull of the weight and the moving joint
decreases, e.g., straight leg raising through a range of 90° with a
loaded weight-boot attached to the foot, and flexion of the gleno-
humeral joint through 90° from lying with a weight held in the
hand.

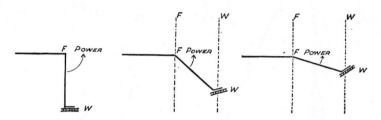

Fig. 5.—Schematic representation of weight resistance applied to the quadriceps extensor
muscle in sitting. The resistance increases from the beginning to the end of the knee-
extension movement because the perpendicular distance between the line of pull of the
weight and the moving joint increases.

When weight resistance is applied to the muscles of the trunk
the same factors hold good. Compare *Trunk raising forward
from fixed lying*, and *Trunk lowering forward from stride standing*.
In the first example the resistance decreases, and in the second it
increases.

Equipment.—The apparatus required is simple and consists
in the main of metal weight-discs of a known poundage, which
are capable of being threaded on to a short, light-weight steel
tube. When the muscles of the lower limbs are exercised the
tube is fitted to a light weight-boot (of alloy), and the weights
secured in place by adjustable collars. When the muscles of the
upper limb are exercised the loaded weight-tube is grasped in
the hand. If very heavy poundages are employed a much heavier
weight-boot (and weight-bar) is generally used.

Trunk movements necessitate the use of either a barbell or
special strap fittings to hold the weights in place.

Relaxation is not so easily obtained as with a weight-and-pulley
circuit, but much can be achieved by the use of special stands on
which the weights are rested at the end of each movement. The
stands also help to prevent joint distraction when a limb is in the
position of rest.

Spring Resistance

Resistance given by helical (long spiral) springs can be useful, but it has two disadvantages. (*a*) It is not physiologically sound, because resistance from springs is always weakest at the beginning of a movement (when the muscles are extended) and strongest at the end of the movement (when the muscles are shortened), and (*b*) it cannot be accurately assessed. Standard helical springs suitable for exercise therapy are calibrated in pounds, the poundage quoted for any given spring representing the pressure exerted when it is extended to its full extent. Therefore the poundage exerted at any point below this level can only be very roughly estimated.

Standard helical springs are obtainable in poundages ranging from 5 to 50 pounds.

Manual Resistance

Self-resistance.—Self-resistance is useful in cases where apparatus is not available, but it cannot be assessed accurately and can only be applied to a limited number of muscle groups. In addition, the patient is not capable of giving or maintaining the amount of resistance which is necessary to strengthen muscles to the degree required for heavy occupations.

Therapist's Resistance.—Resistance by the therapist presents the same difficulties as self-resistance, but it is possible to treat all the main muscle groups of the body.

BASIC PRINCIPLES OF SPECIFIC EXERCISES

All types of specific exercises must conform to three basic principles:—

1. They must be smooth and rhythmical, so that they do not subject muscles and joints to sudden unexpected stresses and strains.

2. They must be based on sound starting positions.

3. They must provide smooth progression from the stage of extreme weakness to the stage of full use against the stresses of normal working conditions.

In addition, all exercises which aim at strengthening weak muscles should provide as wide a range of movement as possible.

PRINCIPLE OF RHYTHM

Muscular contraction must be followed by relaxation, and the relaxation period must be complete and long enough to allow normal circulatory conditions to be restored in the muscle before it begins its next contraction. This principle applies particularly to exercises which are used to redevelop weak muscles after trauma or disuse. It is based on the fact that the efficiency of a muscle depends largely on the condition of its local circulation. If this is good, the breakdown products of contraction are quickly carried away; if it is poor, the products tend to accumulate and produce early fatigue.

To conform to the principle of rhythm in practice the therapist must give as much emphasis to the relaxation period at the end of an exercise as to the actual muscle work itself. Thus, in using an exercise like *Fixed prone lying; Trunk bending backward with Arm turning outward* (*Fig.* 51, p. 47) to strengthen the extensor muscles of the dorsolumbar spine, the following type of coaching technique might be used:—

'Bend back the head—turn out the arms so that the palms face forward—lift the chest from the floor as far as you can . . . . A little more . . . . Now "hold" the position for a moment . . . . Lower the trunk down carefully; let the arms turn in . . . . Now turn the head and flop out completely. Let everything go . . . .' After a few seconds' pause the exercise is repeated.

It is instructive to compare this technique with that often used for the same type of exercise: 'Lift—! Hold the position! Lower . . . . Rest . . . . Lift—!' The instruction for relaxation and the restarting of the exercise almost merge into one another and completely negative the principle of rhythm.

SOUND STARTING POSITION

The starting position from which each exercise is performed should facilitate the work of the muscles, and be suitable for the particular phase of recovery reached by the patient.

Strengthening and Mobilizing.—To strengthen weak muscles or mobilize stiff joints the starting positions of the exercises should be as steady as possible, so as to give the working muscles a firm origin from which to work. The larger the base of support the steadier will be the position of the body. For example, stride standing is steadier than standing, sitting steadier than stride standing, and lying a steadier position than sitting. The nearer the centre of gravity to the base of support, the steadier is the position.

In some instances additional stability is achieved by arranging for the base to be enlarged in the direction of the movement. For example, walk forward standing is a steadier position than stride standing for exercises in which the arms are moved in the sagittal plane, because the movements of the arms cause the centre of gravity of the body to be constantly shifted forward and backward. This is particularly evident when vigorous wide-range arm movements are performed, such as *Arm swinging forward and forward-upward.* In stride standing the compensatory balancing required is achieved not only by essential small movements of the ankle-joints but very often by unnecessary movements in the lumbar spine, with the head and pelvis moving forward and backward alternately.

Developing Co-ordination.—In developing neuromuscular co-ordination the starting position should be chosen so as gradually to increase the difficulty of maintaining the balance, e.g., toe standing and standing with one knee raised forward.

Principle of Progression

The method of progression used depends entirely on whether an exercise is designed to redevelop strength, restore mobility, or redevelop neuromuscular co-ordination (*see* Chap. II, pp. 15–16). One method of progression, however, is common to all types of exercises: progression in time—that is, performing the exercises for increasing periods of time.

Wide-range Movements

Exercises which aim at strengthening muscles should provide as wide a range of movement as possible, and each movement should be taken to its limit. In this way (under minimal stress) it is more likely that all the fibres of the muscle responsible for the movement will be exercised normally. This is important, because it appears from the action of certain muscles that individual groups of muscle-fibres are responsible for particular ranges of movement. In other words, exercising a muscle in part of its range of movement does not necessarily mean that all its fibres will be brought into action. The classic example of this is the vastus medialis muscle, which, under minimal stresses, only contracts during the last 15° of extension of the knee-joint. Therefore, failure to extend the knee to its full extent when exercising the quadriceps extensor muscle group against minimal stresses means that although the vastus lateralis and rectoris femoris sections are exercised, the vastus medialis remains inactive.

CHAPTER II

PROGRESSION OF FREE EXERCISES

1. PROGRESSION IN STRENGTH

PROGRESSION in strength is of great importance in the treatment of injury and disease, because without muscle strength range of movement is useless. On the other hand, strength without range is frequently compatible with full function under the stresses imposed by heavy occupations. Of this Nicoll (1941) says: 'I have seen several instances of men with only 45 degrees of movement at the elbow joint doing work at the coal face while other men with 120 degrees of movement were unable to do so.'

Methods of Progression

There are seven main methods of progressing the strength of free exercises:—

1. By increasing the length of the weight arm of the lever, i.e., arranging the movement so that the centre of gravity of the moving part is further away from the moving joint than before. For example, *Trunk bending backward* from *fixed prone lying* is harder work for the extensors of the dorsolumbar spine and hips when the arms are placed in *neck rest* than when they are by the sides (cf. *Fig.* 47, p. 45, with *Fig.* 51, p. 47); and the exercise is made more difficult still if the arms are held in *stretch* position.

A modification of this type of progression is used in strengthening the spinal rotator muscles in the pelvic rotation exercise shown in *Fig.* 6. In *Fig.* 6 A (*Leg lowering sideways* from *half crook half vertical leg lift lying*) the raised leg acts as a single lever. In *Fig.* 6 B (*slow Leg swinging from side to side* from *vertical leg lift lying*) the combined weight of the two leg levers forms a strong progression on the single-lever system of the first exercise.

It should be noted that the pelvic rotation exercise, *Knee swinging from side to side* from *yard crook lying* (*Fig.* 91, p. 67), is basically a mobility exercise, and is therefore not included in this group.

2. By 'cutting out' the help given to the prime mover muscles by accessory muscles. For example, *Lying; high Leg raising to touch the floor overhead with the toes*, is harder work for the

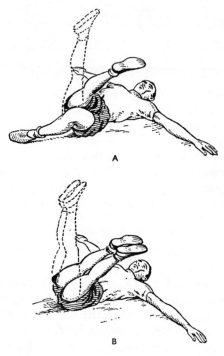

Fig. 6.—Progression in strength: rotator muscles of the dorsal spine. The combined weight of the two-leg lever in B is a strong progression on the single-leg lever of **A**.

abdominal muscles when the arms are in *reach* (*Fig.* 7 B) or *stretch* position, than when they are by the sides (*Fig.* 7 A). In the latter position the accessory flexor muscles of the dorsolumbar spine (latissimus dorsi, teres major, and pectoralis major) come into action to assist the abdominals; they work strongly in inner range, and the first two muscle groups produce extension of the shoulder-joint in addition to spinal flexion. Extension is associated, after some 15°, with shoulder-girdle movement.

N.B.—In general, the most difficult starting position for this exercise is lying with the arms stretched sideways: *yard* (*palms backward*). This is because the position of the arms makes it difficult for the performer to pivot at the dorso-cervical junction, and he has to use his abdominal muscles strongly in an attempt to bring about additional flexion of the dorsolumbar spine.

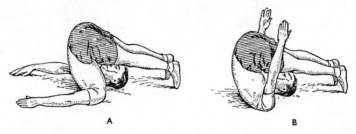

A   B

Fig. 7.—Progression in strength: 'cutting out' the help given to the abdominal muscles by the accessory flexor muscles of the dorsolumbar spine.

3. By increasing the range of movement. For example, spanning performed from *angle hanging* (*Fig.* 8 B) is harder work than when it is performed from the *high reach grasp crook lying* position (*Fig.* 8 A). The exercise is made more difficult still when it is performed from *stretch grasp back support long sitting* (*Fig.* 8 C).

4. By the addition of subsidiary movements to an exercise, so as to increase the work of the main muscle group. For example, *Prone lying; Trunk bending backward with Arm turning outward and single Leg raising backward* (*Fig.* 50, p. 46), is harder work for the extensors of the dorsolumbar spine than the same exercise without the leg movements; and raising both legs backward at the same time (instead of each leg in turn) makes the exercise more difficult still.

5. By using first static and then dynamic muscle work. For example, (*a*) *Half lying; single Quadriceps contractions*, and (*b*) *Half lying* (thighs supported by pillow, with knees flexed to about 45°); *single Knee stretching*.

6. By altering the rhythm of the movement. Slow, controlled movements require more effort from the muscles than the same movements performed at a quicker rate.

7. By altering the effect of gravity on the moving part, i.e., arranging for the movement to be performed with gravity eliminated, and later against the resistance of gravity. Thus, in strengthening the rotators of the dorsal spine: (*a*) *Stride sitting; Trunk turning* and (*b*) *Stride lying; Trunk turning with single Arm carrying across the chest* (*Fig.* 92, p. 68).

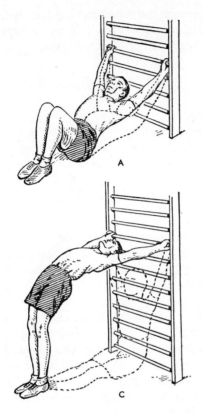

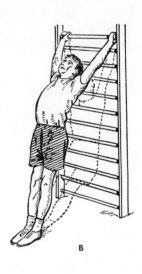

Fig. 8.—Progression in strength: increasing the range of movement in *spanning*.

2. PROGRESSION IN RANGE

From the viewpoint of function, range of movement is undoubtedly secondary in importance to muscle strength. In the restoration of stiff joints after trauma, however, very little headway would be made without employing specific mobility exercises.

Methods of Progression

There are three main methods of progressing the range of free mobility exercises:—

1. By altering the rhythm of the movement. For example, rhythmical swingings are used in place of slow movements.

2. By adding a series of small rhythmical pressing movements to the end of the main movement, e.g., *Stride standing; Trunk*

bending from side to side with rhythmical pressing to three counts in position.

3. By introducing prolonged tension movements. For example, in increasing the range of flexion of a stiff knee-joint, the patient lies on his back with the knee and hip-joints of the affected limb flexed as much as possible without producing pain. He attempts to relax the quadriceps extensor muscle completely, so as to allow the lower leg to hang as a dead weight from the knee. He then contracts the hamstring muscles strongly until the knee-joint is flexed to the limit of pain, 'holds' the position for several seconds, and then allows the hamstrings to relax slowly. This procedure is repeated several times before the knee-joint is extended.

3. PROGRESSION IN CO-ORDINATION

The main methods of progression may be divided into (*a*) those which may be applied to all parts of the body, and (*b*) those which are chiefly applicable to the lower limbs and trunk.

General Methods of Progression

1. Giving movements of the large joints first, and movements of the smaller joints later, e.g., shoulder movements require less co-ordination than finger movements.

2. Increasing the precision with which a controlled movement is performed.

3. Combining movements of different joints, e.g., *Knee full bending with Arm raising sideways.* An extension of this form of progression consists of performing asymmetrical movements, e.g., *opposite Arm swinging sideways and forwards.*

Methods Applicable to Lower Limbs and Trunk

1. Diminishing the size of the accustomed base of support, so that the maintenance of balance becomes a matter of concentrated attention. Generally this is done by (*a*) bringing the feet together (*close standing*); (*b*) raising the heels from the floor (*toe standing*); (*c*) raising one foot from the ground, e.g., *Standing; single Knee raising*; and (*d*) standing or walking on a narrow surface, e.g., balance bench rib or beam.

2. Increasing the difficulties of assuming or maintaining the balance position by (*a*) placing the arms in a higher position (e.g.,

stretch), so as to raise the centre of gravity of the body; (*b*) moving the free joints, and so disturbing the balance (e.g., *Balance half standing* (*beam*); *single Knee raising with Arm raising sideways-upwards*); and (*c*) increasing the height of the apparatus used, which (because of psychological factors) disturbs the equilibrium considerably.

RHYTHMICAL HOPPING AND SKIPPING

Rhythmical hopping and skipping exercises which demand considerable balance are extremely useful in promoting co-ordination. For example (*a*) *Hopping with alternate Toe placing forward and sideways*; (*b*) *Running on the spot with high Knee raising, stopping in position on one leg at a given command*; (*c*) *Skipping: skip jump with rebound, moving forward, backward, right and left, 6 counts in each direction*; and (*d*) *Skipping: hopping with rebound and alternate Knee stretching*.

REFERENCE

NICOLL, E. A. (1941), *Brit. med. J.*, **1**, 501.

CHAPTER III

PROGRESSION OF RESISTED EXERCISES

1. WEIGHT AND WEIGHT-AND-PULLEY EXERCISES

Strength Progression Techniques

IN progressing these exercises the therapist has to bear in mind the fact that although he is aiming at muscle strength and hypertrophy he is dealing in general with weak and atrophied muscles and traumatized joints. Very heavy poundages and comparatively low repetitions—though ideal for boosting the strength of normal muscles—have frequently to be modified considerably, or they may well prove harmful. On the other hand, if the poundages used are kept to a very low figure, with repetitions at a comparatively high level, there is little chance of achieving muscle hypertrophy: the technique will promote the development of endurance rather than the development of strength.

It is difficult, if not impossible, to give a foolproof technique of progression for all conditions and all phases of recovery. It is possible, however, to describe techniques which have been found valuable (and safe) over a considerable period of time.

EARLY TECHNIQUE

It is safe to exercise weak muscles against an *initial* resistance of some 25 per cent of the greatest weight which they can lift ten times in succession without marked discomfort. This ten-times weight is known as the 'Maximum Test Weight', and the other weight as the 'Exercise Weight'. On the first day of treatment the muscles are exercised for one (or two) periods of 4 minutes, each period being halved by a rest pause. Thus the patient exercises for 2 minutes, rests until his muscles feel capable of exercising again, and then exercises for another 2 minutes.

PROGRESSION

Progression in strength is achieved by increasing the weight by a quarter or half a pound when the patient finds that he can do this without undue fatigue or discomfort. (Some degree of fatigue is, of course, unavoidable if the weight is of the poundage necessary to achieve muscle hypertrophy.) The weight increase is continued in this way until the resistance employed is approximately 50 per cent of the maximum test weight (which will also have been increased). The test weight must be checked weekly to ascertain if it can be increased—an important aim of treatment.

Progression in time is brought about by increasing the exercise time by 1 minute each day until the patient is exercising for 15 minutes before the rest pause, and 15 minutes after it. The length of the rest pause depends on the degree of muscle fatigue. As previously stated, the exercise periods may be given once or twice daily, e.g., morning and afternoon.

More Advanced Technique

This technique may be used as a progression on that previously described (when the muscles have reached a satisfactory state of redevelopment), and in cases where a more strenuous initial exercise technique can be tolerated.

Thus, at the start of the exercise session, the maximum test weight is lifted ten times; the exercise weight is then lifted for the appropriate time, complete with rest pause. The test weight is then lifted again ten times.

It is important to note that although the patient may not be able finally to accomplish ten correctly performed lifts, he should be encouraged to make the number of lifts that are possible. Unless this is done maximum muscle hypertrophy will not result. Expert supervision and care are most important in this type of training; an enthusiastic patient may attempt too much and bring about muscular strain or joint effusion.

Technique of Exercise

The movements must be performed smoothly and fairly slowly in such a way that the muscles work concentrically, statically, and then eccentrically. Thus, in strengthening the quadriceps extensor muscle from a firm sitting position on a fixation bench, the patient extends the knee-joint to its full extent, 'holds' it in this position for a moment, and then allows it to return to the starting position. After a brief relaxation pause the movement is repeated. (*See Fig.* 2, p. 3, which shows weight-and-pulley resistance applied to the quadriceps.)

In exercising the muscles of the limbs it is usual to limit resistance to the affected limb only. When the limbs are equal in strength, however, the sound limb may be exercised against resistance, also. In practice this is seldom necessary, because the sound limb will be exercised adequately during other aspects of the patient's rehabilitation programme: during sessions devoted to specific and general exercises and recreational therapy.

Assessing Muscle Strength

In redeveloping weak muscles it is important to test periodically the maximum test weight of the corresponding sound muscle group, so that the relative weakness of the affected muscle group may be ascertained, and a 'target' established for the patient. The result is expressed as a fraction: Left/Right =20 lb./9 lb. in the case of a weak right quadriceps extensor muscle. In dealing with the trunk muscles, where this type of comparison is not possible, a known standard is determined by testing out a number of normal subjects.

The maximum test weights of the affected and corresponding sound muscle groups should be recorded weekly and plotted as a graph. These tests not only form a reliable guide to progress but are extremely instructive.

Each time the tests are made the same weight apparatus or weight-and-pulley circuit should be used. This is particularly important when using pulley circuits, because the frictional resistance offered by individual pulley sheaves varies considerably. The same precaution applies when weights and weight-and-pulley circuits are used for exercise purposes.

Making a Test

In assessing the maximum test weight of a muscle group it is important for the patient to avoid trying out too many different poundages before arriving at the correct one, or the muscles will become so fatigued by this preliminary work that it will be almost impossible to make an accurate test. A useful method of determining the test weight is for the therapist to load the patient's muscles with a weight which he considers to be a reasonable poundage for the purposes of the test, and then ask him to make a *small* movement against its resistance. In this way the patient can try the effect of the weight on his muscles without using them sufficiently to fatigue them. If he finds the weight is too much, or too little (bearing in mind a series of ten repetitions), the poundage is adjusted accordingly and the test repeated. When the patient feels that the correct weight has been found, he tries the ten full movements against it. If the patient and the therapist are satisfied after this that the weight is the right one, no further tests are made; if they are not satisfied with the result, the muscles are allowed to rest until they are ready for exercise again and a further test is made.

Other Methods of Resistance Training

The training methods described in the previous section are based on those originally formulated by Nicoll and Colson in 1940, as part of a pioneer scheme of medical rehabilitation for injured miners in this country (Nicoll, 1941 and 1943). Later, other methods of resistance training (based on the heavy resistance techniques used by bodybuilders and weight-lifters) were developed from time to time. Three main systems, known by the names of their originators, are in use today: (*a*) De Lorme and Watkins (1951) technique; (*b*) Zinovieff (1951) (Oxford technique); and (*c*) McQueen (1954) technique.

HEAVY-RESISTANCE SYSTEMS

The heavy-resistance techniques are mainly intended for use with weights, although they may be equally well used with weight-and-pulley circuits.

Common to the three techniques is the Ten Repetition Maximum (10 R.M.): the maximum poundage which can be lifted by the weak muscle group for ten repetitions only. For example, in determining the 10 R.M. of a weak quadriceps extensor muscle, the patient assumes a sound starting position on a fixation bench, with a weight-boot strapped to his foot, and observes the following schedule: Starting with the weight of the weight-boot, and increasing by small amounts (e.g., 1–5 lb.), he lifts each weight ten repetitions at a natural speed and without rests between lifts. That weight which requires maximum exertion to perform ten repetitions is thus determined.

De Lorme and Watkins 'Fractional' Technique

In this system the 10 R.M. resistance is *increased* gradually over a limited series of repetitions. Thus:—

> 1st set: 10 lifts with half 10 R.M.
> 2nd set: 10 lifts with three-quarters 10 R.M.
> 3rd set: 10 lifts with 10 R.M.

In this way, some 30 repetitions of the 10 R.M. are carried out daily, 4 times per week (total of 120 lifts). Each week the 10 R.M. is progressed.

Zinovieff (Oxford Technique)

In this system the 10 R.M. resistance is gradually *decreased* over a comparatively wide series of repetitions. Thus:—

> 1st set: 10 lifts with 10 R.M.
> 2nd set: 10 lifts with 10 R.M. *subtracting* 1 lb.
> 3rd set: 10 lifts with 10 R.M. *subtracting* 2 lb.
> 4th set: 10 lifts with 10 R.M. *subtracting* 3 lb.
> 5th set: 10 lifts with 10 R.M. *subtracting* 4 lb.
> 6th set: 10 lifts with 10 R.M. *subtracting* 5 lb.
> 7th set: 10 lifts with 10 R.M. *subtracting* 6 lb.
> 8th set: 10 lifts with 10 R.M. *subtracting* 7 lb.
> 9th set: 10 lifts with 10 R.M. *subtracting* 8 lb.
> 10th set: 10 lifts with 10 R.M. *subtracting* 9 lb.

In this manner, some 100 resistance repetitions are performed daily, 5 times per week (total of 500 lifts). Each day an attempt is made to progress the 10 R.M.

McQueen Technique

In this system the 10 R.M. resistance is *maintained* (without addition or subtraction) over a limited series of lifts. Thus:—

> 1st set: 10 lifts with 10 R.M.
> 2nd set: 10 lifts with 10 R.M.
> 3rd set: 10 lifts with 10 R.M.

In this way, some 30 repetitions of the 10 R.M. are performed 3 times weekly (total of 90 lifts). Progress is achieved by attempting to increase the 10 R.M. weekly.

LIMITATION OF HEAVY-RESISTANCE SYSTEMS.—Heavy-resistance techniques are undoubtedly capable of producing muscle hypertrophy and strength, but must be used with great care in exercise therapy. On the whole, they are more applicable to the late phase of recovery from injury or disease than to any other stage. If used in the earlier phases considerable modification is frequently necessary to avoid muscle strain and joint reaction.

2. SPRING AND MANUAL RESISTANCE

Progression in Strength

SPRING RESISTANCE

Accurate and precise progression in strength is not possible because of the nature of spring resistance (p. 7). An overall and very approximate degree of progression is achieved by increasing the poundage of the spring or springs employed, e.g., replacing a 10-lb. spring by a 15- or 20-lb. spring, or increasing the number of springs arranged in parallel.

Tension in Springs.—When arranging spring resistance, it is important to see that the spring or springs are slightly stretched in the starting position, so that resistance is offered to the muscles from the start to the finish of the movement. If the spring or springs are not under tension in the starting position the initial part of the patient's movement will be expended in taking up the slack.

MANUAL RESISTANCE

Only a very rough and approximate degree of progression is possible, whether the resistance is given by the therapist or the patient.

REFERENCES

DE LORME, T. L., and WATKINS, A. L. (1951), *Progressive Resistance Exercises—Techniques and Medical Application.* New York: Appleton-Century-Crofts.
McQUEEN, I. (1954), *Brit. med. J.*, **2**, 1193.
NICOLL, E. A. (1941), *Ibid*, **1**, 501.
— — (1943), *Ibid.*, **1**, 747.
ZINOVIEFF, A. (1951), *Brit. J. phys. Med. ind. Hyg.*, **14**, 129.

PART II

PROGRESSIVE EXERCISES

INTRODUCTION

THE free exercises listed here are arranged progressively in terms of strength and mobility, as described in Chapter II (pp. 11–16), and include movements for all parts of the body.

In arranging the trunk and neck exercises (where a very wide range of exercises has to be covered), each section devoted to a particular muscle group is divided into (*a*) Static Exercises and (*b*) Dynamic Exercises, together with a brief analysis of the main types of movement.

Grading.—All the exercises listed are grouped under three main headings: Early, Intermediate, and Advanced. In turn, each group is divided (wherever feasible) into two or more grades.

Numbers prefixing the exercises indicate progression throughout the various grades. Where more than one exercise of the same type is listed in a grade, the number is followed by A, B, or C to indicate this (*see* p. 47, Intermediate Exercises for Spinal Extensors).

CHAPTER IV

HEAD AND NECK EXERCISES

HEAD and neck exercises provide work for the muscles which activate the atlanto-occipital joints and the joints of the cervical spine. The exercises given here have been classified in relation to the individual muscle groups.

Starting Positions.—Many types of starting positions are used for head and neck exercises, but those most useful for remedial work are sitting, low grasp sitting (*Fig.* 9), and reach grasp sitting (*Fig.* 10). Crook sitting and cross sitting (*Figs.* 11 and 12) are often used in the treatment of small children. The low grasp and reach grasp sitting positions are valuable when head side bending and head turning exercises are performed, because the shoulders are fixed.

In this chapter the sitting position has been used when describing exercises which may be performed from it or any of its suitable modifications.

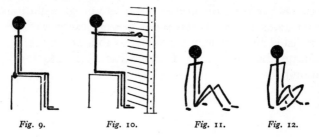

Fig. 9.   *Fig. 10.*   *Fig. 11.*   *Fig. 12.*

FLEXORS OF HEAD AND NECK

Types of Dynamic Exercises

HEAD ON TRUNK.—Three main groups of exercises are classified here:—

1. Flexion of the head and neck from lying and crook lying.

Example: *Yard (palms backward) lying; Head bending forward* (*Fig.* 13).

2. Part-range (from and to midline) extension and flexion of the head and neck from sitting (*see* p. 24).

Example: *Sitting; Head bending backward.*

3. Full-range flexion and extension of the head and neck from the high lying position with the head unsupported.

Example: *High lying (plinth: head unsupported); Head bending forward and backward, and return to starting position (Fig. 14).*

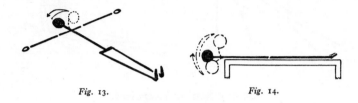

Fig. 13.   Fig. 14.

Strengthening Exercises

Elementary.—
Grade 1.
1. Sitting; Head bending backward.

Grade 2.
1. No progression.
2. Yard (palms backward) lying; Head bending forward. (*See Fig.* 13.)

Intermediate.—
Grade 1.
1. No progression.
2. High lying (plinth: head unsupported); Head bending forward and backward, and return to starting position. (*See Fig.* 14.)

EXTENSORS OF HEAD AND NECK

Types of Static Exercises

1. ATTEMPTED MOVEMENT.—Attempted movement of the head and neck from lying and crook lying without movement of the joints.

Example : *Lying; Head pressing backward.*

2. FIXATION OF HEAD AND NECK.—Stabilization of the head and neck in the Body raising type of exercise from a suitable lying position.

Example: *Stride lying (head supported by partner); 'Log raising' by partner (Fig. 15).*

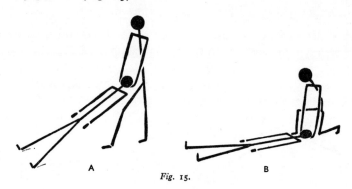

Fig. 15.

Strengthening Exercises
Elementary: No. 1, above; *Advanced:* No. 2, above.

Types of Dynamic Exercises

1. HEAD ON TRUNK.—Two main groups of exercises are classified here:—

a. Part-range (from and to midline) flexion and extension of the head and neck from sitting (*see* p. 24), or extension of the head and neck from prone lying.

Example: (i) *Sitting; Head bending forward.*

(ii) *Forehead rest prone lying; Head bending backward.*

b. Full-range flexion and extension of the head and neck from prone kneeling.

Example: *Prone kneeling; Head bending forward and backward, and return to starting position (Fig. 16).*

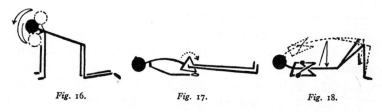

Fig. 16.   *Fig. 17.*   *Fig. 18.*

2. TRUNK ON HEAD.—This group includes the Chest raising and Wrestler's Bridge types of exercises; they are performed from

such starting positions as lying, crook lying, and stride crook lying.

Example: (i) *Lying; Chest raising (Fig.* 17).

(ii) *Arm cross stride crook lying (head on mat); press up to high Wrestler's Bridge (Fig.* 18).

Strengthening Exercises

Elementary.—
Grade 1.

1. Sitting; Head bending forward.

Grade 2.

1. Prone kneeling; Head bending forward and backward, and return to starting position. (*See Fig.* 16, p. 26.)

2. Forehead rest prone lying; Head bending backward.

3. Lying; Chest raising. (*See Fig.* 17, p. 26.)

Intermediate.—
Grade 1.

1 and 2. No progressions.

3. Crook lying; Chest raising.

Grade 2.

1 and 2. No progressions.

3. Neck rest crook lying; Chest raising.

Advanced.—
Grade 1.

1 and 2. No progressions.

3. Arm cross stride crook lying (head on mat); press up to high Wrestler's Bridge. (*See Fig.* 18, p. 26.)

Grade 2.

1 and 2. No progressions.

3. Arm cross stride lying (head on mat); press up to low Wrestler's Bridge (*Fig.* 19).

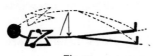

Fig. 19.

Mobilizing Exercises

Elementary.—

Grade 1.

1. Sitting; Head dropping forward and stretching upward.

2. Sitting; Head nodding forward (1–2), followed by stretching upward (3–4).

Grade 2.

1. Prone kneeling; Head bending forward, and bending backward with rhythmical pressing to a given count, followed by return to starting position.

1A. Prone kneeling; Head bending forward and backward continuously.

2. Prone kneeling; Head dropping forward and bending backward.

3. Forehead rest prone lying; Head bending backward with rhythmical pressing to a given count.

FLEXORS AND EXTENSORS OF HEAD AND NECK
Types of Dynamic Exercises

HEAD ON TRUNK.—Three main groups of exercises are classified here:—

1. Full-range flexion and extension of the head and neck from crook side lying.

Example: *Crook side lying; Head bending forward and backward, and return to starting position.*

2. Part-range (from and to midline) or full-range flexion and extension of the head and neck from sitting (*see* p. 24).

Example: *Sitting; Head bending forward to press the chin gently against the chest, followed by Head bending backward, and return to starting position.*

3. Straightening of the cervical concavity with slight flexion of the atlanto-occipital joints, followed by flexion of the neck with extension of the atlanto-occipital joints (Chin indrawing and poking forward). The movements are usually taken from sitting (*see* p. 24).

Strengthening Exercises

Elementary.—

Grade 1.

1. Crook side lying; Head bending forward and backward, and return to starting position.

Grade 2.

1. No progression.

2. Sitting; Head bending forward to press the chin gently against the chest, and Head stretching upward.

3. Sitting; Head bending forward to press the chin gently against the chest, followed by Head bending backward, and return to starting position.

4. Sitting; Chin indrawing and poking forward, and return to starting position.

Mobilizing Exercises

Elementary.—

Grade 1.

1. Crook side lying; Head bending forward and backward continuously.

Grade 2.

1. No progression.

LATERAL FLEXORS OF HEAD AND NECK

Types of Dynamic Exercises

HEAD ON TRUNK.—Lateral flexion of the head and neck from lying, crook side lying, and sitting (*see* p. 24).

Example: (i) *Crook lying; Head bending sideways.*

(ii) *Crook side lying (head resting on pillow); Head bending sideways (Fig.* 20).

(iii) *Sitting; Head bending from side to side.*

Strengthening Exercises

Elementary.—

Grade 1.

1. Crook lying; Head bending sideways.

Grade 2.

1. Sitting; Head bending sideways.

Intermediate.—

Grade 1.

1. Crook side lying (head resting on pillow); Head bending sideways. (*See Fig.* 20, p. 30.)

Grade 2.

1. Crook side lying (head touching supporting surface); Head bending sideways (*Fig.* 21).

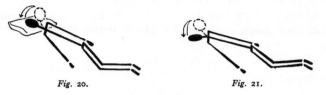

Fig. 20.   Fig. 21.

Mobilizing Exercises

Elementary.—

Grade 1.

1. Crook lying; Head bending from side to side.

Grade 2.

1. Sitting; Head bending from side to side.

2. Sitting; Head bending sideways with rhythmical pressing to a given count.

ROTATORS OF HEAD AND NECK

Types of Dynamic Exercises

HEAD ON TRUNK.—Rotation of the head and neck from lying, crook lying, and sitting (p. 24).

Example: (i) *Crook lying; Head turning.*

(ii) *Sitting; Head turning from side to side.*

Strengthening Exercises

Elementary.—

Grade 1.

1. Crook lying; Head turning.

1A. Sitting; Head turning.

Mobilizing Exercises

Elementary.—

Grade 1.

1. Crook lying; Head turning from side to side.

1A. Sitting; Head turning from side to side.

Grade 2.

1A. Sitting; Head turning with rhythmical pressing to a given count.

CIRCUMDUCTORS OF HEAD AND NECK

Types of Dynamic Exercises

HEAD ON TRUNK.—Circumduction of the head and neck from sitting (*see* p. 24) and prone kneeling.

Mobilizing Exercises

Elementary.—

Grade 1.

1. Sitting; Head rolling.

Grade 2.

1. Prone kneeling; Head rolling.

Chapter V

TRUNK EXERCISES

Trunk exercises provide work for the spinal muscles which act on the dorsolumbar spine and pelvis; many of the exercises also activate the muscles of the hips, cervical spine, and atlanto-occipital joints.

The exercises given here have been classified in relation to the individual muscle groups of the dorsolumbar spine.

FLEXORS OF THE SPINE

Types of Static Exercises

1. Abdominal Retraction.—Retraction of the abdominal muscles from such starting positions as crook lying, prone lying, sitting, and standing.

Example: *Crook lying; Abdominal contractions.*

2. Leg or Legs on Trunk.—In this group of exercises the hips are flexed in turn, or together, through a given range of movement. The abdominal muscles act statically to prevent the pelvis from being tilted forward by the contraction of the hip flexors of the moving leg or legs. When the legs are moved in turn the hip extensors of the resting leg act statically with the abdominal muscles to fix the pelvis.

Four main types of exercises are classified here. They are taken from such starting positions as lying, standing, and hanging.

a. Flexion of the hip and knee of one leg almost to the full extent.*

Example: *Lying; single high Knee raising (Fig. 22).*

b. Flexion of one or both hips up to 90° with flexion of the knee or knees.

Example: *Lying; single Knee raising.*

---

* In the average subject flexion of one hip (with the knee well flexed) through the final degrees of movement is associated with small range backward tilting of the pelvis. Flexion of the hip should, therefore, not be taken to its full extent if a pure static action of the abdominal muscles is required.

c. Flexion of one hip through 45°, with the knee extended.

Example: *Lying; single Leg raising through 45°.*

d. Flexion of the hips to 45° with the knees extended.

Example: *Stretch grasp back toward standing (wall bars); Leg raising to 45°.*

3. TRUNK (SPINE STRAIGHT) ON LEGS.—

a. Trunk lowering backward and raising from fixed inclined long sitting with the spine held straight. The hips are alternately extended and flexed through a range of 35–65°.

Example: *Wing fixed inclined long sitting (wall bar stool); Trunk lowering backward through 45° (Fig. 23).*

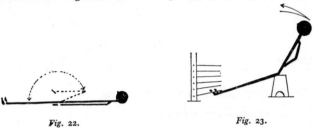

Fig. 22.   Fig. 23.

During the raising and lowering movements the abdominal muscles act statically to maintain the straight position of the spine.

b. Trunk raising and lowering from fixed lying, with the spine held straight. The hips are alternately flexed and extended through a range of about 90°.

Example: *Wing fixed lying; Trunk raising (Fig. 24).*

During the raising and lowering movements the abdominal muscles act statically to maintain the straight position of the trunk.

4. HEAD ON TRUNK.—Head bending forward from lying and crook lying. The abdominal muscles act statically to fix the origin of the scalene muscles and the sternomastoid muscles.

Example: *Crook lying; Head bending forward.*

Head bending forward is often combined with hip flexion movements to increase the static action of the abdominal muscles.

Example: *Lying; Head bending forward with single high Knee raising.*

5. Arm Bending from Prone Falling Position and its Modifications.—During the exercise the abdominal muscles act statically to prevent gravity from tilting the pelvis forward and exaggerating the lumbar concavity.

Example: *Inclined prone falling (hands on beam); Arm bending (Fig. 25).*

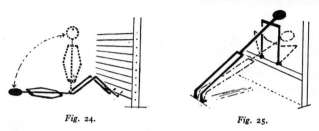

Fig. 24.   Fig. 25.

Strengthening Exercises

Elementary.—

Grade 1.

1. Crook lying; Abdominal contractions.

2. Lying; single Knee raising.

3. Lying; single high Knee raising. (*See Fig. 22, p. 33.*)

4. Lying; single Leg raising to 45°.

5. Lying; single high Knee raising, Leg stretching forward to 45°, and slow lowering.

6. Crook lying; Head bending forward.

7. Lying; Head bending forward with single high Knee raising.

8. Low grasp fixed inclined long sitting (hands grasping front edge of wall-bar stool); Trunk lowering backward through 35°.

Grade 2.

1. Prone lying; Abdominal contractions.

2. Lying; Knee raising (*Fig. 26*).

3. Lying; cycling.

4. Lying; alternate Leg raising through 45°.

4A. Lying; single Leg raising to 45°, followed by Leg raising to 5°.

5 and 6. No progressions.

7. Yard (palms backward) lying; Head bending forward with single Leg raising through 45°.

8. Wing fixed inclined long sitting (wall bar stool or balance bench); Trunk lowering backward through 35°.

9. Inclined prone falling (hands on beam); Arm bending. (*See Fig.* 25, p. 34.)

Intermediate.—
Grade 1.

1. No progression.

2. Stretch grasp back toward standing (wall bars); Knee raising.

3. No progression.

4. Lying; Leg raising through 45°.

4A–7. No progressions.

8. Wing or fist bend fixed inclined long sitting (wall bar stool); Trunk lowering backward through 45°. (*See Fig.* 23, p. 33.)

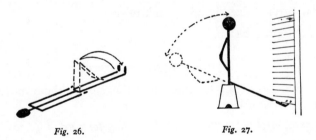

Fig. 26.　　　　　Fig. 27.

9. Inclined prone falling (hands on beam); Arm bending. (*See Fig.* 25, p. 34.)

Grade 2.

1–7. No progressions.

8. Wing or neck rest fixed inclined long sitting (wall bar stool); Trunk lowering backward through 45–65° (*Fig.* 27).

8A. Wing fixed lying; Trunk raising. (*See Fig.* 24, p. 34.)

9. Prone falling; Arm bending (*Fig.* 28).

Advanced.—

Grade 1.

1–7. No progressions.

8. Stretch fixed inclined long sitting (wall bar stool); Trunk lowering backward through 45–65°.

8A. Neck rest fixed lying; Trunk raising.

9. Horizontal prone falling; Arm bending (*Fig.* 29).

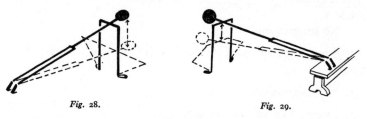

Fig. 28.   Fig. 29.

Grade 2.

1–7. No progressions.

8. Stretch fixed crook sitting; Trunk lowering backward to the floor.

8A. Stretch fixed lying; Trunk raising.

9. No progression.

Types of Dynamic Exercises

1. SPINE ON PELVIS.—Flexion of the spine without movements of the pelvis or legs.

Example: *Lying; upper Trunk bending forward* (*Fig.* 30).

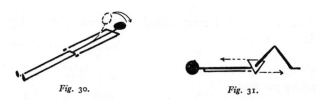

Fig. 30.   Fig. 31.

2. PELVIS AND LUMBAR SPINE ON UPPER TRUNK AND LEGS.— Pelvis tilting backward, the abdominal muscles acting with the hip extensors.

Example: *Crook lying; Pelvis tilting backward* (*Fig.* 31).

3. LEGS ON PELVIS: PELVIS AND LUMBAR SPINE ON UPPER TRUNK.—Full flexion of the hips and knees, or flexion of the hips with the knees extended, combined with flexion of the dorsolumbar spine.

Example: (i) *Lying; high Knee raising (Fig. 32).*

(ii) *Lying; high Leg raising to touch the floor behind the head with the toes (Fig. 33).*

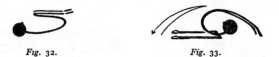

Fig. 32.   Fig. 33.

A modification of this type of exercise consists of circling on rings or ropes. The extensors of the dorsolumbar spine work to a small extent, but the main emphasis of the exercise is on the abdominal and heaving muscles.

Example: *Stretch grasp standing (rings); circling and return circling with straight legs (Fig. 34).*

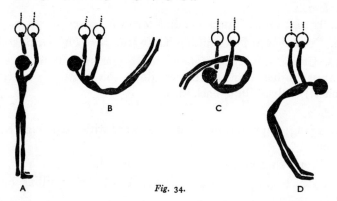

A   B   C   Fig. 34.   D

4. SPINE ON PELVIS: PELVIS ON LEGS.—Flexion of the spine and hips, the legs being fixed by apparatus or living support.

Example: *Wing fixed crook lying; Trunk bending forward (Fig. 35).*

5. COMBINED MOVEMENTS OF TRUNK AND LEG OR LEGS.— Flexion of the spine combined with knee-raising movements; the legs are either moved together, or one at a time.

Example: (i) *Lying; high Knee raising, followed by over-pressure with the hands, and upper Trunk bending forward (Fig. 36).*

(ii) *Lying; upper Trunk bending forward with single high Knee raising.*

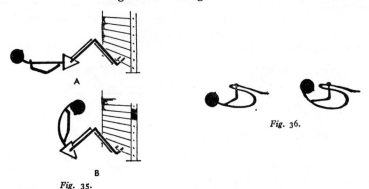

Fig. 36.

Fig. 35.

Strengthening Exercises

Elementary.—

Grade 1.

1. Lying; upper Trunk bending forward. (*See Fig.* 30, p. 36.)

2. Crook lying; Pelvis tilting backward. (*See Fig.* 31, p. 36.)

2A. Crook side lying (under hand grasping front edge of mattress, other hand pressing down on mattress in front of chest); Pelvis tilting backward.

Grade 2.

1. Lying; upper Trunk bending forward with single high Knee raising.

2. Prone kneeling; Pelvis tilting backward.

2A. Reach grasp kneel sitting (wall bars); Pelvis tilting backward.

2B. Reach grasp sitting (wall bars); Pelvis tilting backward.

2C. Reach grasp standing (wall bars); Pelvis tilting backward.

3. Lying; high Knee raising. (*See Fig.* 32, p. 37.)

Intermediate.—

Grade 1.

1. Fixed crook lying; Trunk bending forward with assistance from the arms.

2–2C. No progressions.

3. Lying; high Knee raising, followed by overpressure with the hands, and upper Trunk bending forward. (*See Fig.* 36, p. 38.)

Grade 2.

1. Wing fixed crook lying; Trunk bending forward. (*See Fig.* 35, p. 38.)

2–2C. No progressions.

3. Lying (wall bars behind head); high Knee raising and stretching to touch a low bar with the toes.

4. Heave grasp walk forward standing (rings); circling and return circling with bent knees, touching the floor with the feet at the end of the forward circling movement.* (*See Fig.* 34, p. 37.)

Advanced.—
Grade 1.

1. Neck rest fixed crook lying; Trunk bending forward.

2–2C. No progressions.

3. Lying; high Leg raising to touch the floor behind the head with the toes. (*See Fig.* 33, p. 37.)

4. Heave grasp walk forward standing (rings); circling and return circling with straight legs, touching the floor with the feet at the end of the forward circling movement.* (*See Fig.* 34, p. 37.)

5. Stretch grasp back toward standing (wall bars); high Knee raising.

Grade 2.

1–2C. No progressions.

3. Reach (or stretch) lying; high Leg raising to touch the floor behind the head with the toes.

4. Stretch grasp standing (rings); circling and return circling with straight legs. (*See Fig.* 34, p. 37.)

5. Hanging (wall bars); high Knee raising.

---

* The extensor muscles of the dorsolumbar spine act to a small extent, but the main emphasis of the exercise is on the abdominal muscles and depressors of the arms.

Grade 3.

1–2C. No progressions.

3. Yard (palms backward) lying; high Leg raising to touch the floor behind the head with the toes.

4. Inward grasp hanging (rings); circling and return circling with straight legs.*

5. Hanging (wall bars); high Leg raising.

EXTENSORS OF THE SPINE

Types of Static Exercises

1. LEG ON TRUNK.—Raising each leg backward, in turn, from prone lying, so that the hip joint is extended about 15°. The extensors of the dorsolumbar spine and the hip flexors of the stationary leg act statically to prevent the pelvis from being tilted backward by the contraction of the hip extensors of the moving leg.

Example: *Forehead rest prone lying; single slight Leg raising backward.*

When hip extension is taken beyond 15° the pelvis tilts forward, because of the tension exerted on the ilio-femoral ligament. The extensors of the dorsolumbar spine then act dynamically.

2. TRUNK (SPINE STRAIGHT) ON LEGS.—Trunk lowering and raising from such starting positions as sitting, stride standing, and fixed high thigh support across prone lying. The trunk is kept straight while the hips are alternately flexed and extended. The extensors of the dorsolumbar spine act statically throughout the lowering and raising movements to prevent gravity from flexing the spine.

The range of the hip movements varies in the different starting positions, as outlined below.

a. Sitting and stride sitting. The forward lowering movement is limited by the apposition of the soft structures of the thighs and abdomen.

Example: *Wing stride sitting; Trunk lowering forward (Fig.* 37).

---

* The extensor muscles of the dorsolumbar spine act to a small extent, but the main emphasis of the exercise is on the abdominal muscles and the depressors of the arms.

b. Standing and stride standing. The forward lowering movement is taken as far as the length of the hamstring muscles allows.

Example: *Wing stride standing; Trunk lowering forward.*

c. Fixed high thigh support across prone lying. The position is usually taken over two balance benches, one being placed on top of the other. Trunk lowering forward is limited by the contact of the head with the floor.

Example: *Wing fixed high thigh support across prone lying (balance benches, 2 high); Trunk lowering forward (Fig. 38).*

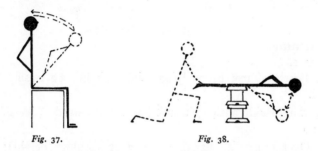

Fig. 37.   Fig. 38.

This type of movement is usually introduced by a ' holding ' exercise.

Example: *Wing fixed high thigh support across prone lying (balance benches, 2 high); position holding.*

3. Arm Bending from Fall Hanging Position or its Modifications.—During the exercise the extensors of the dorsolumbar spine act statically to maintain a straight position of the trunk and to prevent gravity from flexing it.

Example: *Over grasp fall hanging (beam at shoulder height); Arm bending (Fig. 39).*

4. Fallout Forward Exercises.—The exercises are performed with or without arm movements. The extensors of the dorsolumbar spine act statically to counteract gravity and to maintain a straight position of the spine. Unless the exercises are performed with perfect control the extensors will be used dynamically.

Example: *Wing standing; fallout forward, left Foot forward, right Foot forward (Fig. 40).*

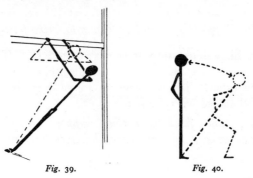

Fig. 39.   *Fig. 40.*

Strengthening Exercises

Elementary.—

Grade 1.

1. Forehead rest prone lying; single slight Leg raising backward.

2. Wing stride sitting; Trunk lowering forward. (*See Fig.* 37, p. 41.)

3. Over grasp fall hanging (beam at shoulder height); Arm bending. (*See Fig.* 39.)

Grade 2.

1. No progression.

2. Wing stride standing; Trunk lowering forward.

3. Over grasp fall hanging (beam below shoulder height); Arm bending.

Intermediate.—

Grade 1.

1. No progression.

2. Fist bend stride standing; Trunk lowering forward.

2A. Wing fixed high thigh support across prone lying (balance benches, 2 high); position holding.

3. Over grasp fall hanging (beam below shoulder height); Arm bending with single Leg raising.

4. Wing standing; fallout forward, left Foot forward, right Foot forward. (*See Fig.* 40.)

Grade 2.

  1. No progression.

  2. Neck rest stride standing; Trunk lowering forward.

  2A. Wing fixed high thigh support across prone lying (balance benches, 2 high); Trunk lowering forward. (*See Fig.* 38, p. 41.)

  3. Over grasp horizontal fall hanging (beam and living support); Arm bending (*Fig.* 41).

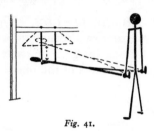

Fig. 41.

  4. Across bend standing; fallout forward, left Foot forward, right Foot forward, with Arm flinging.

Advanced.—
Grade 1.

  1. No progression.

  2. Stretch stride standing; Trunk lowering forward.

  2A. Neck rest fixed high thigh support across prone lying (balance benches, 2 high); Trunk lowering forward. (*See Fig.* 38, p. 41.)

  3. Over grasp horizontal fall hanging (beam and balance benches, 2 high); Arm bending with single Leg raising.

  4. Fist bend standing; fallout forward, left Foot forward, right Foot forward, with Arm stretching forward.

Grade 2.

  1–4. No progressions.

Types of Dynamic Exercises

  1. PELVIS AND LUMBAR SPINE ON UPPER TRUNK AND LEGS.— Pelvis tilting forward, the extensors of the dorsolumbar spine acting with the flexors of the hips.

  Example: *Crook lying; Pelvis tilting forward* (*Fig.* 42).

2. LEG ON PELVIS: PELVIS AND LUMBAR SPINE ON UPPER TRUNK.—Raising in turn each leg backward beyond 15° from prone lying or reach grasp standing. The ilio-femoral ligament of the moving hip-joint checks hip extension after about 15°; to extend the leg further the pelvis is tilted forward as far as possible by the extensors of the dorsolumbar spine and the flexors of the hip of the stationary leg.

Example: *Forehead rest prone lying; single Leg raising backward.*

3. TRUNK (SPINE ARCHED) ON LEGS.—This group includes Chest raising and preparatory Spanning exercises which are taken from lying and crook lying. The extensors of the dorsolumbar spine act with the flexors of the hips.

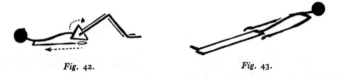

Fig. 42.   *Fig. 43.*

Example: (i) *Lying; Chest raising (Fig. 43).*

(ii) *High reach grasp lying (wall bars: hands grasping 5th or 6th bar from floor); spanning (Fig. 44).*

In these exercises crook lying is used as a progression on lying; it places the hip flexors in a shortened position, and so reduces their ability to raise the pelvis and lumbar spine from the floor.

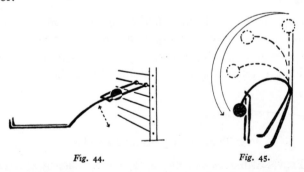

Fig. 44.   *Fig. 45.*

4. SPINE ON PELVIS: PELVIS ON LEGS.—In this group of exercises the extensors of the dorsolumbar spine are used with the extensors of the hips. There are three main types of exercises:—

a. Extension of the spine and hips from lax stoop stride sitting or standing, or any other suitable starting position, to bring the trunk to the erect position.

Example: *Lax stoop back lean stride standing (heels 12–15 in. in front of wall or upright); Trunk stretching ' vertebra by vertebra' (Fig. 45).*

b. As the previous type of exercise, but the trunk is uncurled to the stoop position.

Example: *Fist bend lax stoop kneel sitting; Trunk stretching forward to stoop position with Arm stretching sideways (Fig. 46).*

c. Extension of the dorsolumbar spine and hips from prone lying with the legs fixed.

Example: *Neck rest fixed prone lying; Trunk bending backward (Fig. 47).*

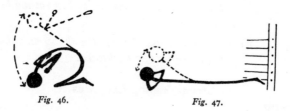

Fig. 46.   Fig. 47.

5. SPINE ON PELVIS.—Extension of the dorsolumbar spine from prone lying. The extensors of the dorsolumbar spine are used dynamically; the extensors of the hips act statically to fix the pelvis.

Example: *Prone lying; Trunk bending backward with Arm turning outward (Fig. 48).*

6. COMBINED MOVEMENTS OF LEGS OR LEG ON PELVIS WITH EXTENSION OF SPINE.—In these exercises the extensors of the dorsolumbar spine are used with the extensors of the hips. There are two main groups of exercises:—

a. Spanning exercises and similar movements.

Example: (i) *Angle hanging (wall bars); spanning (Fig. 49).*

(ii) *Arm cross stride crook lying (head on mat); press up to high Wrestler's Bridge. (See Fig. 18, p. 26.)*

b. Extension of the dorsolumbar spine from prone lying combined with extension of the lower limbs; the limbs are either moved in turn, or together.

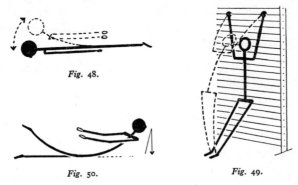

Fig. 48.

Fig. 50.   Fig. 49.

Example: (i) *Prone lying; Trunk bending backward with Arm turning outward and single Leg raising backward (Fig. 50).*

(ii) *Neck rest prone lying; Trunk bending backward with Leg raising backward.*

Strengthening Exercises

Elementary.—
Grade 1.

1. Lying; Chest raising. (*See Fig.* 43, p. 44.)

2. Crook lying; Pelvis tilting forward. (*See Fig.* 42, p. 44.)

2A. Crook side lying (under hand grasping front edge of mattress, other hand pressing down on mattress in front of chest); Pelvis tilting forward.

3. Forehead rest prone lying; single Leg raising backward.

4. Lax stoop stride sitting (hands on thighs, and lower part of sacrum in contact with wall or upright); Trunk stretching 'vertebra by vertebra' with assistance from arms.

5. Lax stoop kneel sitting (palms on floor with elbows bent); Trunk stretching forward to stoop position with Elbow stretching.

Grade 2.

1. Crook lying; Chest raising.

2. Reach grasp kneel sitting (wall bars); Pelvis tilting forward.

2A. Reach grasp sitting (wall bars); Pelvis tilting forward.

2B. Reach grasp standing (wall bars); Pelvis tilting forward.

3. Fixed prone lying; Trunk bending backward with Arm turning outward (*Fig.* 51).

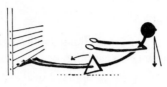

Fig. 51.

3A. Prone lying; Trunk bending backward with Arm turning outward. (*See Fig.* 48, p. 46.)

4. Lax stoop back lean stride standing (heels 12–15 in. in front of wall or upright); Trunk stretching 'vertebra by vertebra'. (*See Fig.* 45, p. 44.)

4A. Lax stoop kneel sitting (hands clasped behind back); Trunk stretching with unclasping of hands and Arm turning outward.

5. As above, but Trunk is stretched forward to stoop position.

6. Crook lying; Pelvis raising. (*See Fig.* 112, p. 84.)

Intermediate.—
Grade 1.

1. Neck rest crook lying; Chest raising.

1A. High reach grasp lying (wall bars: hands grasping 5th or 6th bar from floor); spanning. (*See Fig.* 44, p. 44.)

2. No progression.

3. Neck rest fixed prone lying; Trunk bending backward. (*See Fig.* 47, p. 45.)

3A. Neck rest prone lying; Trunk bending backward.

3B. Prone lying; Trunk bending backward with Arm turning outward and single Leg raising backward. (*See Fig.* 50, p. 46.)

4. As Exercise 4 above, but arms in neck rest.

4A. Neck rest lax stoop kneel sitting; Trunk stretching 'vertebra by vertebra'.

5. Fist bend lax stoop kneel sitting; Trunk stretching forward to stoop position with Arm stretching sideways. (*See Fig.* 46, p. 45.)

6. No progression.

Grade 2.

1. No progression.

1A. High reach grasp crook lying (wall bars: hands grasping 5th or 6th bar from floor); spanning.

1B. Stretch grasp back support kneel sitting (wall bars); spanning (*Fig.* 52).

2. No progression.

3. Head rest fixed prone lying; Trunk bending backward.

3A. Prone lying; Trunk bending backward with Arm turning outward and Leg raising backward.

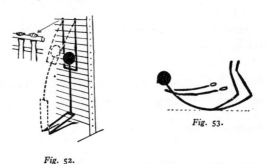

Fig. 52.

Fig. 53.

3B. Stride prone lying; Trunk bending backward combined with Arm turning outward, Knee bending and Leg raising backward, so as to bring the heels together (*Fig.* 53).

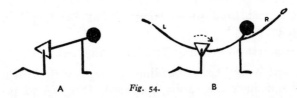

A   *Fig.* 54.   B

3C. Prone kneeling; single Arm raising forward-upward with opposite Leg stretching and raising backward (*Fig.* 54).

4. No progression.

4A. Fist bend lax stoop leg backward stretch half kneel sitting; Trunk stretching to arch position (*Fig.* 55).

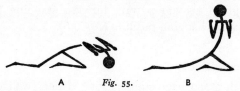

A   *Fig. 55.*   B

5. Lax stoop stride standing (hands clasped behind neck, elbows forward); Trunk stretching forward with Elbow parting to neck rest position.

6. No progression.

Advanced.—
Grade 1.

1. No progression.

1A. Angle hanging (wall bars); spanning. (*See Fig.* 49, p. 46.)

1B–2. No progressions.

3. Stretch fixed prone lying; Trunk bending backward.

3A. Neck rest prone lying; Trunk bending backward with Leg raising backward.

3B–4. No progressions.

4A. As Exercise 4A Intermediate, Grade 2, but arms in neck rest position. (*See Fig.* 55.)

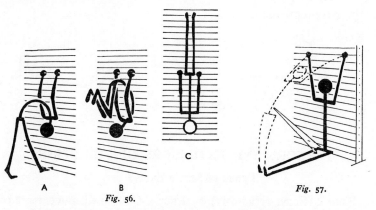

A   B   *Fig. 57.*
Fig. 56.

5. Lax stoop stride standing; Trunk stretching forward with Arm stretching forward-upward to stretch position.

6. Arm cross stride lying (head on mat); press up to high Wrestler's Bridge. (*See Fig.* 19, p. 27.)

7. Drag grasp lax stoop walk forward standing (wall bars); assuming reverse hanging position (*Fig.* 56).

Grade 2.

1. No progression.

1A. Stretch grasp back support long sitting (wall bars); spanning (*Fig.* 57).

1B–2. No progressions.

3. Neck rest lax stoop fixed high thigh support across prone lying (balance benches, 2 high); Trunk stretching to arch position (*Fig.* 58).

3A. Stretch prone lying; Trunk bending backward with Leg raising backward.

3B–4. No progressions.

4A. As Exercise 4A, Intermediate, Grade 2, but arms in stretch position. (*See Fig.* 55.)

5. No progression.

6. Arm cross stride lying (head on mat); press up to low Wrestler's Bridge. (*See Fig.* 19, p. 28.)

6A. Stride crook lying (palms on floor behind shoulders, elbows forward); press up to the Crab (*Fig.* 59).

7. No progression.

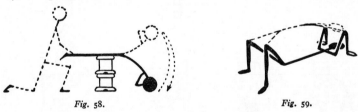

Fig. 58.   Fig. 59.

FLEXORS AND EXTENSORS OF THE SPINE
Types of Static Exercises

TRUNK (SPINE STRAIGHT) ON LEGS.—Combined movements of trunk lowering backward and forward (pp. 33 and 40) are taken from fixed inclined long sitting with the knees slightly flexed.

The spinal flexors and extensors act statically to keep the spine straight, while the hips are alternately extended and flexed.

The backward lowering movements are taken through a range of 35–65°; the forward lowering movements are limited by the tension of the hamstring muscles. During trunk lowering backward and raising the spinal flexors are used statically; the spinal extensors act statically as the trunk is lowered forward and raised.

Example: *Wing fixed inclined long sitting (wall bar stool); Trunk lowering backward through 65°, raising and lowering forward, and return to starting position (Fig. 60).*

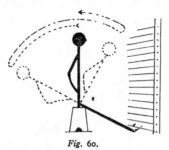

Fig. 60.

Strengthening Exercises

Trunk lowering forward movements are added to the trunk lowering backward exercises which are performed from fixed inclined long sitting (pp. 34–36). *See* example above.

Types of Dynamic Exercises

1. PELVIS AND LUMBAR SPINE ON UPPER TRUNK AND LEGS.— Pelvis tilting forward and backward from such starting positions as crook lying, prone kneeling, and reach grasp sitting. The extensors and flexors of the dorsolumbar spine act with the hip flexors and extensors.

Example: *Crook lying; Pelvis tilting forward and backward.* (*See Figs.* 42 and 31, pp. 44 and 36.)

2. COMBINED MOVEMENTS OF TRUNK AND LEG OR LEGS.—

a. Simultaneous movement of trunk and each leg in turn. The spine is flexed and extended in prone kneeling, the movements being accompanied by flexion and extension of each leg.

Example: *Prone kneeling; single high Knee raising with Head bending forward, followed by Leg stretching and raising backward with Head bending backward, and return to starting position (Fig.* 61).

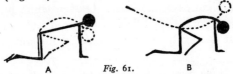

A   *Fig.* 61.   B

b. Simultaneous movement of trunk and both legs. This group of exercises includes:—

i. Flexion and extension of the spine, hips, and knees in side lying.

Example: *Side lying; Trunk bending forward with high Knee raising, followed by Trunk stretching backward with Leg stretching and carrying backward (Fig.* 62).

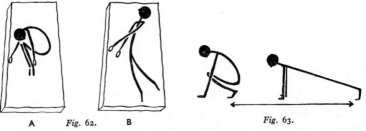

A   *Fig.* 62.   B   *Fig.* 63.

ii. Jumping the feet rhythmically backward and forward between crouch sitting and prone falling (*Fig.* 63).

iii. Nest Hang exercises in rings.

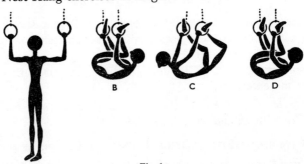

A   *Fig.* 64.

Example: *Hanging from hands and feet (rings); Nest Hang (Fig.* 64).

iv. Circling exercises at the beam.

Example: *Under grasp walk forward standing (beam at head height); circling forward-upward and downward-forward with straight legs (Fig. 65).*

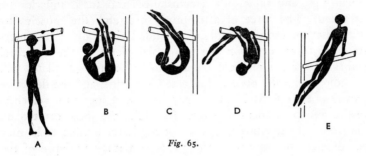

Fig. 65.

3. SPINE ON PELVIS: PELVIS ON LEGS.—Two main groups of exercises are classified here:—

a. Flexion and extension exercises of the spine and hips which incorporate rhythmical pressing or over-stressing movements in full flexion. The exercises are often considered to be of use in increasing flexion of the dorsolumbar spine and in 'stretching' the hamstring muscles. The usual starting positions for the movements are stride standing, long sitting, and fixed toward standing at the wall bars. (*See Fig.* 67, p. 54.)

Example: i. *Stride standing; Trunk bending forward-downward with rhythmical pressing to beat the floor (1–3), followed by slow Trunk stretching upward (4–6) (Fig. 66).*

ii. *Fist bend long sitting; Trunk bending forward with Arm stretching forward to reach the toes, or beyond them, with 3 presses.*

iii. *Fixed toward standing (wall bars); Trunk bending forward to grasp the ankle of the raised leg— over-stressing of Trunk bending—and slow stretching upward (Fig. 67).*

All the rhythmical pressing and over-stressing trunk flexion exercises have been deliberately omitted from the list of mobility exercises in this section, because they are considered by orthopædic surgeons to be wholly pernicious. *The exercises never, on*

3

any occasion, do any good, and they are calculated to do the utmost harm to the spine, even when the hamstrings do not seriously limit hip flexion.

A large number of people have congenital shortening of the hamstrings, and under no circumstances can these muscles be stretched. The force of attempting to stretch the muscles by spinal flexion exercises will be expended either upon the intervertebral disks, or upon the epiphysial plates of the vertebral bodies. In the adolescent damage to the epiphysial plates will be radiographically observed as osteochondritis, and the defective growth of the epiphysial plates may cause wedging of the vertebral bodies and permanent damage. In adults the force exerted on the fronts of the annulus fibrosis of the lower lumbar disks may be sufficient to rupture it and produce a frank prolapse of the nucleus pulposus.

b. Wide range *strengthening* exercises for the flexors and extensors of the spine and hips, which are taken from fixed inclined long sitting (*see Fig.* 68). The trunk is flexed to the *lax stoop* position, fully extended, and then returned to the erect position.

> Example: *Wing fixed inclined long sitting (balance bench); Trunk bending forward to lax stoop position, followed by Trunk stretching upward, lowering, and bending backward to touch the floor with the head, and return to starting position (Fig. 68).*

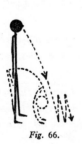 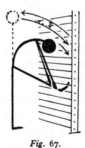 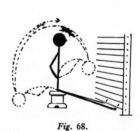

Fig. 66.   *Fig. 67.*   *Fig. 68.*

Strengthening Exercises

Elementary.—
Grade 1.
No exercises.

Grade 2.

1. Prone kneeling; single high Knee raising with Head bending forward, followed by Leg stretching and raising backward with Head bending backward, and return to starting position. (*See Fig.* 61, p. 52.)

Intermediate.—
Grade 1.

1. No progression.

2. Under grasp walk forward standing (beam at head height); circling forward-upward and downward-forward with bent knees.* (*See Fig.* 65, p. 53, which shows the exercise performed with straight knees.)

Grade 2.

1. No progression.

2. Under grasp walk forward standing (beam at head height); circling forward-upward and downward-forward with straight legs. (*See Fig.* 65, p. 53.)

3. Low grasp fixed inclined long sitting (balance bench); Trunk bending forward to lax stoop position, followed by Trunk stretching upward, lowering and bending backward to touch the floor with the head, and return to starting position. (*See Fig.* 68, p. 54, which shows a different starting position.)

Advanced.—
Grade 1.

1. No progression.

2. Stretch under grasp standing (beam); circling forward-upward and downward-forward with straight legs. (*See Fig.* 65, p. 53, which shows an easier starting position.)

3. Wing fixed inclined long sitting (balance bench); Trunk bending forward to lax stoop position, followed by Trunk stretching upward, lowering and bending backward to touch the floor with the head, and return to starting position. (*See Fig.* 68, p. 54.)

Grade 2.

1. No progression.

---

* For introductory circling exercises at the beam, *see* Technical Points, p. 58.

2. Under grasp hanging (beam); circling forward-upward and downward-forward with straight legs. (*See Fig.* 65, p. 53, which shows an easier starting position.)

3. As Exercise 3, Grade 1, but with arms in neck rest position.

Mobilizing Exercises

Elementary.—
Grade 1.

1. Crook lying; Pelvis tilting forward and backward. (*See Figs.* 42 and 31, pp. 44 and 36.)

1A. Crook side lying (under hand grasping front edge of mattress, other hand pressing down on mattress in front of chest); Pelvis tilting forward and backward.

2. Side lying; Trunk bending forward with high Knee raising, followed by Trunk bending backward with Leg stretching and carrying backward. (*See Fig.* 62, p. 52.)

2A. As the previous exercise, but during each trunk arching movement only one leg is carried back to the full extent.

Grade 2.

1. Prone kneeling; Pelvis tilting forward and backward with Head bending backward and forward (*Fig.* 69).

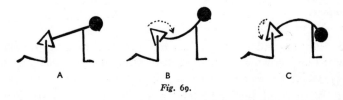

A　　　　　　　　B　　　　　　　　C
Fig. 69.

1A. Reach grasp kneel sitting (wall bars); Pelvis tilting forward and backward.

1B. Reach grasp sitting (wall bars); Pelvis tilting forward and backward.

1C. Reach grasp standing (wall bars); Pelvis tilting forward and backward.

2–2A. No progressions.

Intermediate.—

Grade 1.

1. Wide lax stretch (palms downward) lax stoop kneel sitting; Pluto sniffing (*Fig.* 70).

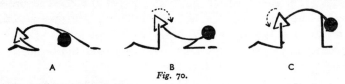

A   B   C
Fig. 70.

2–2A. No progressions.

3. Hanging from hands and feet (rings or ropes); Nest Hang. (*See Fig.* 64, p. 52.)

4. Crouch sitting; alternating between prone falling and crouch sitting by jumping the Feet rhythmically backward and forward (1–6). (*See Fig.* 63, p. 52.)

Grade 2.

1–2A. No progressions.

3. Hanging from hands and feet (rings); Nest Hang with single Leg raising backward (*Fig.* 71).

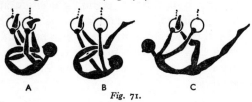

A   B   C
Fig. 71.

Advanced.—

Grade 1.

1–2A. No progressions.

3. Hanging from hands and feet (rings); half Nest Hang (*Fig.* 72).

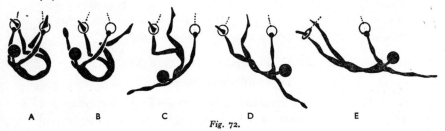

A   B   C   D   E
Fig. 72.

TECHNICAL POINTS

INTRODUCTORY EXERCISES TO CIRCLING ON THE BEAM

1. BEAM ARRANGED AT HIP LEVEL.—The subject takes up an under grasp curtsy sitting position, so that the chest is pressed against the beam and the feet are under it. He then practises throwing the legs up to the beam with bent knees. Later, he attempts to straighten the knees and pull over the beam to the standing position on the other side.

2. BEAM A LITTLE UNDER HIP HEIGHT.—The subject stands close to the beam, and grasps it with the fingers behind and the thumbs in front, so that the hands touch the thighs. He then leans over the beam as far as possible, simultaneously bringing the chin up to the chest and looking at the knees; he then bends the knees and brings the heels up to the seat, which allows the weight of the upper part of the body to carry the legs over the beam. The body should be kept in this flexed position until the feet touch the floor.

3. USING TWO BEAMS: LOWER BEAM PLACED AT CHEST LEVEL, AND UPPER BEAM ABOUT TWO FEET ABOVE IT.—The subject takes up the under grasp walk forward standing position at the lower beam. He throws the legs up and gets the heels behind the upper beam; he then presses with the heels and bends the arms and circles up on the lower beam to the balance hanging position. In circling forward-downward he bends the hip and knee joints as much as possible.

USE OF SUPPORTERS

Until the subject has acquired a good circling technique two supporters should stand on either side of him to give him confidence. Support is most often required when the subject changes his grasp before extending the body, and the assistants' hands should be placed under the shoulders and legs. It is also a wise precaution to put an agility mattress or mat under the beam in case the subject should accidentally lose his grasp.

LATERAL FLEXORS OF THE SPINE

Types of Static Exercises

1. TRUNK (SPINE STRAIGHT) ON LEG.—Trunk lowering and raising sideways from standing or thigh support side toward

standing by abducting and adducting the hip joint of one leg, the other leg being raised and lowered sideways with the trunk. Throughout the exercise the lateral flexors of the spine on the upper side act statically to keep the spine straight and to prevent gravity from side flexing it.

Example: *Side toward standing (wall bar stool); Trunk lowering sideways to place the hand on the stool with single Leg raising sideways (Fig. 73).*

2. LATERAL MOVEMENTS OF THE ARM AND/OR LEG FROM SIDE FALLING POSITION OR ITS MODIFICATIONS.—During the exercises the lateral flexors of the dorsolumbar spine on the lower side act statically to keep the trunk straight and to prevent it from sagging.

Example: *Side falling; single Leg raising sideways (Fig. 74).*

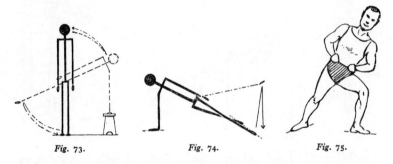

Fig. 73.   Fig. 74.   Fig. 75.

3. FALLOUT OUTWARD EXERCISES.—The exercises are performed with or without arm movements. The lateral flexors of the dorsolumbar spine of the upper side act statically to keep the spine straight and to prevent it from bending towards the side of the forward leg. Unless the exercises are performed with perfect control the lateral flexors will be used dynamically.

Example: *Wing standing; fallout outward, left and right (Fig. 75).*

Strengthening Exercises

Elementary.—

Grade 1.

1. Side toward standing (wall bar stool); Trunk lowering sideways to place the hand on the stool with single Leg raising sideways. (*See Fig. 73.*)

2. Inclined side falling (hand on wall bar stool); single Leg raising sideways.

Grade 2.

1. Half stretch side toward standing (wall bar stool); Trunk lowering sideways to place the free hand on the stool with single Leg raising sideways.

2. Side falling; single Leg raising sideways. (*See Fig.* 74, p. 59.)

Intermediate.—

Grade 1.

1. Wing thigh support side toward standing (beam); Trunk lowering sideways with single Leg raising sideways (*Fig.* 76).

2. Half fist bend side falling; single Leg raising sideways with single Arm stretching sideways-upward.

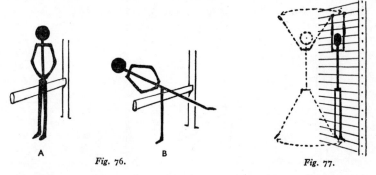

Fig. 76. Fig. 77.

3. Wing standing; fallout outward, left and right. (*See Fig.* 75, p. 59.)

4. Stretch grasp high toward toe standing (wall bars); assuming Star position (*Fig.* 77).

Grade 2.

1. Half stretch half wing thigh support side toward standing (beam); Trunk lowering sideways with single Leg raising sideways.

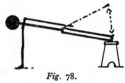

Fig. 78.

2. Horizontal side falling; single Leg raising sideways (*Fig.* 78).

3. Fist bend standing; fallout outward, left and right, with Arm stretching upward.

4. No progression.

Advanced.—
Grade 1.

1. Stretch side toward standing (wall bars); Trunk lowering sideways to grasp the bars with single Leg raising sideways.

2. Half fist bend horizontal side falling; single Leg raising sideways with single Arm stretching sideways-upward.

3–4. No progressions.

Grade 2.

No progressions.

Types of Dynamic Exercises

1. SPINE ON PELVIS.—Lateral flexion of the spine from a starting position which fixes the pelvis, such as ride sitting, stride sitting, and foot support side toward standing (*see* Fixation of Pelvis, p. 66).

Example: (i) *Stride sitting; Trunk bending sideways.*

(ii) *Ride sitting (chair: thighs gripping chair back); Trunk bending from side to side (Fig. 79).*

(iii) *Half neck rest foot support side toward standing (wall bars); Trunk bending sideways towards the bars with rhythmical pressing to 3 counts (Fig. 80).*

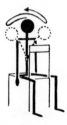
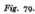
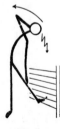
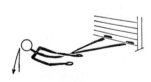

Fig. 79.   Fig. 80.   Fig. 81.

2. SPINE ON PELVIS: PELVIS ON LEGS.—Lateral flexion of the trunk from a starting position which allows lateral pelvic tilting to occur, such as stride standing, stride lying, and fixed side

lying. The lateral flexors of the dorsolumbar spine act with the hip abductors and adductors.

Example: (i) *Stride standing; Trunk bending from side to side.*

(ii) *Stride lying; Trunk bending sideways.*

(iii) *Fixed side lying (one leg slightly in front of other); Trunk bending sideways (Fig. 81).*

3. LEGS ON PELVIS: PELVIS AND LUMBAR SPINE ON UPPER TRUNK.—Leg raising sideways or leg swinging from side to side from hanging; this group of exercises includes leg lowering sideways from reverse hanging. The lateral flexors of the dorsolumbar spine act with the hip abductors and adductors.

Example: (i) *Hanging (wall bars); Leg raising sideways (Fig. 82).*

(ii) *Over grasp hanging (beam); Arm walking sideways with Leg swinging from side to side (Fig. 83).*

4. PELVIS AND LUMBAR SPINE ON UPPER TRUNK.—Hip updrawing from such starting positions as heave grasp lying and reach grasp standing. The pelvis is tilted sideways by the combined action of the lateral flexors of the dorsolumbar spine of the side of the raised hip, and the hip abductors of the opposite side.

Example: *Reach grasp standing (wall bars); Hip updrawing (Fig. 84).*

This group of exercises includes lateral pelvic tilting from side to side; the usual starting positions for these movements are reach grasp kneel sitting and reach grasp standing.

Example: *Reach grasp kneel sitting (wall bars); Pelvis tilting from side to side.*

5. SIMULTANEOUS MOVEMENT OF TRUNK AND ONE LEG.—Lateral flexion of the spine combined with either *Hip updrawing* or *single Leg carrying sideways* of the side to which the trunk is moved. The movements are performed in lying.

Example: (i) *Lying; Trunk bending sideways with Hip updrawing of the same side.*

(ii) *Lying; Trunk bending sideways with single Leg carrying to the same side.*

6. PELVIS LOWERING AND RAISING FROM SIDE FALLING POSITION.—Pelvis lowering and raising from side falling by combined movements of lateral flexion of the dorsolumbar spine

and hip abduction and adduction. The lateral flexors of the
dorsolumbar spine on the underneath side of the trunk act with
the hip abductors of the underneath leg and the hip adductors
of the uppermost leg.

> Example: *Side falling (one leg slightly in front of other)*; *Pelvis
> lowering to touch supporting surface, raising as high as possible,
> and return to starting position (Fig. 85).*

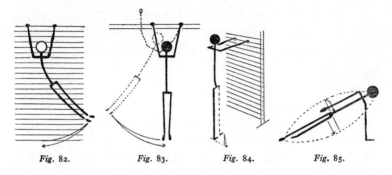

Fig. 82.   Fig. 83.   Fig. 84.   Fig. 85.

Strengthening Exercises

Elementary.—

Grade 1.

   1. Stride lying; Trunk bending sideways.

   2. Heave grasp lying (mattress) or lying (hands grasping sides
of mattress); Hip updrawing. (*See Fig.* 84.)

   3. Stride sitting; Trunk bending sideways.

Grade 2.

   1. Lying; Trunk bending sideways with single Leg carrying
to the same side.

   1A. Lying; Trunk bending sideways with Hip updrawing of
the same side.

   2. Reach grasp standing (wall bars); Hip updrawing. (*See
Fig.* 84.)

   3. Neck rest stride sitting; Trunk bending sideways.

   4. Neck rest stride standing; Trunk bending sideways.

Intermediate.—

Grade 1.

   1 and 1A. No progressions.

2. Reach grasp high half standing (wall bars and stool); Hip sinking, updrawing, and lowering to starting position.

3. Stretch ride sitting (chair: thighs gripping chair back); Trunk bending sideways.

4. Stretch stride standing; Trunk bending sideways.

Grade 2.

1–4. No progressions.

5. Side falling (one leg slightly in front of other); Pelvis lowering to touch supporting surface, raising as high as possible, and return to starting position. (*See Fig.* 85, p. 63.)

Advanced.—
Grade 1.

1–5. No progressions.

6. Fixed side lying (one leg slightly in front of other); Trunk bending sideways. (*See Fig.* 81, p. 61.)

7. Reverse hanging (wall bars); Leg lowering sideways (*Fig.* 86, p. 66).*

Grade 2.

1–5. No progressions.

6. Half neck rest fixed side lying (one leg slightly in front of other); Trunk bending sideways.

7. Hanging (wall bars); Leg raising sideways. (*See Fig.* 82, p. 63.)*

Mobilizing Exercises
Elementary.—
Grade 1.

1. Stride lying; Trunk bending from side to side.

Grade 2.

1. Stride standing; Trunk bending from side to side.

2. Ride sitting (chair: thighs gripping chair back); Trunk bending from side to side. (*See Fig.* 79, p. 61.)

3. Reach grasp kneel sitting (wall bars); Pelvis tilting from side to side.

---

* Leg lowering sideways from reverse hanging is easier for the working muscles than leg raising sideways from hanging. The reverse hanging position, however, is a difficult one for the average patient to maintain; for this reason leg raising sideways from hanging is often used before the other exercise.

Intermediate.—
Grade 1.

1. Neck rest stride standing; Trunk bending from side to side.

1A. Stride standing; Trunk bending from side to side with rhythmical pressing to 3 counts in position.

2. Neck rest ride sitting (chair: thighs gripping chair back); Trunk bending from side to side.

2A. Ride sitting (chair: thighs gripping chair back); Trunk bending from side to side with rhythmical pressing to 3 counts in position.

3. No progression.

4. Stride standing; Trunk bending sideways with single Arm (of opposite side) swinging forward-downward-sideways-upward, the Trunk being bent to the side during the sideways-upward swing of the arm.

5. Half neck rest foot support side toward standing (wall bars); Trunk bending sideways towards the bars with rhythmical pressing to a given count. (*See Fig.* 80, p. 61.)

6. Half neck rest leg sideways stretch half kneeling; Trunk bending sideways with rhythmical pressing to a given count (*Fig.* 87).

Grade 2.

1. Head rest stride standing; Trunk bending from side to side.

1A–4. No progressions.

5. Wing fixed side toward standing (wall bars); Trunk bending sideways towards the bars with rhythmical pressing to 3 counts, and bending away from the bars to 3 slow counts. (*See Fig.* 88.)

6. No progression.

7. Over grasp hanging (beam); Arm walking sideways with Leg swinging from side to side. (*See Fig.* 83, p. 63.)

Advanced.—
Grade 1.

1. Lax stretch stride standing; Trunk bending from side to side.

1A–4. No progressions.

5. As Exercise 5, Intermediate, Grade 2, but arms in neck rest (*Fig.* 88).

6. No progression.

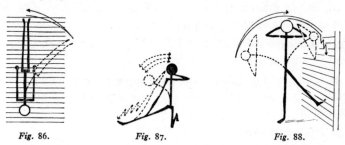

Fig. 86.   Fig. 87.   Fig. 88.

Fixation of Pelvis during Lateral Flexion of Spine

The pelvis is securely fixed in the following positions:—

1. *Ride sitting* on a chair, or a balance bench, with the thighs gripping the chair back, or the legs gripping the bench sides. (*See Fig.* 79, p. 61 and *Fig.* 89.)

2. *High ride sitting*, with the legs gripping the high plinth.

The pelvis is also firmly fixed in positions where one leg is supported, with the hips fully abducted; such positions include *foot support* (or *fixed*) *side toward standing*, and *leg sideways stretch half kneeling*. (*See Fig.* 80, p. 61 and *Fig.* 87.) The pelvis is less securely fixed in *stride sitting*.

ROTATORS OF THE SPINE

Types of Dynamic Exercises

1. SPINE ON PELVIS.—Rotation of the spine from a starting position which fixes the pelvis, such as ride sitting and prone kneeling (*see* Fixation of Pelvis, p. 70).

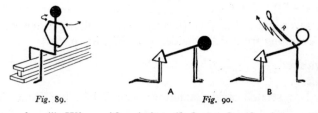

Fig. 89.   A   Fig. 90.   B

Example: (i) *Wing ride sitting (balance bench: legs gripping bench sides); Trunk turning (Fig.* 89).

(ii) *Prone kneeling; Trunk turning with single Arm swinging sideways and rhythmical pressing to 3 counts (Fig. 90).*

2. LEGS, PELVIS, AND LUMBAR SPINE ON UPPER TRUNK.—Rotation of the trunk by moving the pelvis and legs together, the upper trunk being the fixed point.

Example: *Yard (palms backward) crook lying; Knee swinging from side to side (Fig. 91).*

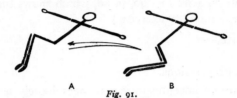

Fig. 91.

3. SPINE ON PELVIS: PELVIS ON LEGS.—Rotation of the trunk from a starting position which allows hip rotation, such as stride standing, standing, and stride lying.

Example: *Stride standing; Trunk turning from side to side with Arm swinging loosely at the sides.*

4. PELVIS AND LUMBAR SPINE ON UPPER TRUNK AND LEGS.—Pelvic rotation from a starting position which allows hip rotation and fixes the upper trunk and legs.

Example: *Reach grasp close standing (wall bars); Pelvis turning.*

Strengthening Exercises

Elementary.—

Grade 1.

1. Wing ride sitting (balance bench: thighs gripping bench sides); Trunk turning. (*See Fig.* 89, p. 66.)

2. Wing stride sitting; Trunk turning.

3. Stride standing; Trunk turning.

4. Reach grasp close standing (wall bars); Pelvis turning.

Grade 2.

1 and 2. No progressions.

3. Stride lying; Trunk turning with single Arm carrying across the chest (*Fig.* 92).

4. Heave grasp lying (wall bars); Pelvis turning.

4A. Crook lying; Pelvis raising, turning, and lowering.

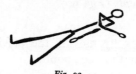

Fig. 92.

5. Prone kneeling; slow Trunk turning with single Arm raising sideways. (*See Fig.* 90, p. 66, which shows the movement performed as a mobility exercise.)

Intermediate.—

Grade 1.

1–4A. No progressions.

5. Turn prone kneeling (one arm bent loosely across chest); slow Trunk turning with single Arm raising sideways. (*See Fig.* 90, p. 66, which shows the movement performed as a mobility exercise.)

Grade 2.

1–5. No progressions.

6. Yard (palms backward) half crook half vertical leg lift lying; Leg lowering sideways (*Fig.* 93).

Advanced.—

Grade 1.

1–5. No progressions.

6. Yard (palms backward) vertical leg lift lying; slow Leg swinging from side to side (*Fig.* 94).

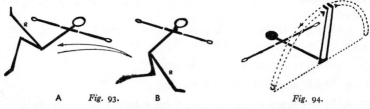

A   *Fig.* 93.   B   *Fig.* 94.

Mobilizing Exercises

Elementary.—

Grade 1.

1. Arm cross ride sitting (chair: thighs gripping chair back); Trunk turning from side to side.

2. Stride standing; Trunk turning from side to side with Arms swinging loosely at the sides.

Grade 2.

1. Across bend ride sitting (chair: thighs gripping chair back); Trunk turning from side to side with alternate Arm flinging.

2. Half lumbar rest stride standing; single Arm swinging forward, and sideways with Trunk turning.

3. Yard (palms backward) crook lying; Knee swinging from side to side. (*See Fig.* 91, p. 67.)

4. Prone kneeling; Trunk turning with single Arm swinging sideways. (*See Fig.* 90, p. 66.)

Intermediate.—

Grade 1.

1. Arm cross ride sitting (chair: thighs gripping chair back); Trunk turning from side to side with rhythmical pressing to 3 counts in position.

2. Stride standing; Trunk turning from side to side with Arm swinging loosely at the sides and rhythmical pressing to 3 counts in position.

3. No progression.

4. Turn prone kneeling (one arm bent loosely across chest); Trunk turning with single Arm swinging sideways and rhythmical pressing to 3 counts (*Fig.* 95).

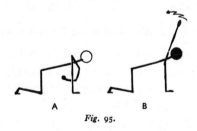

A   B

Fig. 95.

5. Reach half kneeling; Trunk turning with single Arm swinging sideways and rhythmical pressing to a given count.

Grade 2.

1–5. No progressions.

6. Over grasp fixed stride fall hanging (beam: feet fixed by living support); Trunk turning with single Arm swinging sideways to touch floor. (*See Fig.* 97.)

Advanced.—
Grade 1.

1–3. No progressions.

4. Lax reach stoop stride standing; Trunk turning from side to side with alternate Arm swinging sideways and across the chest (*Fig.* 96).

5. No progression.

6. Over grasp horizontal fall hanging (beam and living support: beam at such a height that hand cannot touch floor if grasp of one hand is released); Trunk turning with single Arm swinging sideways (*Fig.* 97).

Grade 2.

No progressions.

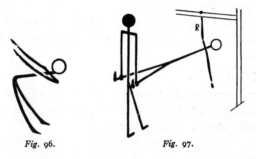

Fig. 96.　　　　*Fig.* 97.

Fixation of Pelvis during Spinal Rotation

The pelvis is securely fixed in the following positions:—

1. *Ride sitting* on a chair, or a balance bench, with the thighs gripping the chair back, or the legs gripping the bench sides. (*See Figs.* 79 and 89, pp. 61 and 66.)

2. *High ride sitting*, with the legs gripping the high plinth.

The pelvis is also well fixed in *prone kneeling* (*see Fig.* 90, p. 66). *Cross sitting* and *kneel sitting* give good fixation of the pelvis, but adults usually find these positions difficult to maintain. *Sitting, stride sitting, long sitting,* and *crook sitting* provide some fixation of the pelvis.

COMBINED EXERCISES FOR THE ROTATORS, FLEXORS, AND EXTENSORS

Types of Dynamic Exercises

Only the main types of combined exercises have been classified here. All the exercises are based on the following sequence of movement—Spine on Pelvis: Pelvis on Legs.

1. WORKING FLEXORS AND ROTATORS OF SPINE WITH HIP ROTATORS.—Flexion and rotation of the trunk, without flexion of the hips, from lying and stride lying.

Example: *Stride lying; upper Trunk bending forward with turning and single Arm carrying across the chest (Fig. 98).*

2. WORKING FLEXORS AND ROTATORS OF SPINE AND HIPS.— Flexion and rotation of the spine and hips from fixed lying and fixed crook lying.

Example: *Neck rest fixed crook lying; Trunk bending forward with turning (Fig. 99).*

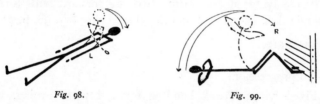

Fig. 98.　　　　Fig. 99.

3. WORKING EXTENSORS AND ROTATORS OF SPINE WITH HIP EXTENSORS.—Extension and rotation of the spine, with extension of the hips, from a lax stoop position which prevents pelvic rotation. (*See* Fixation of Pelvis, p. 70.)

Example: *Fist bend lax stoop kneel sitting; Trunk stretching 'vertebra by vertebra' with turning (Fig. 100).*

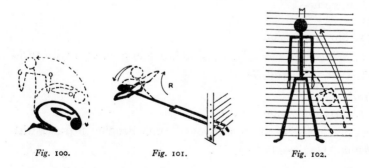

Fig. 100.　　　　Fig. 101.　　　　Fig. 102.

4. WORKING EXTENSORS AND ROTATORS OF SPINE AND HIPS.—
Extension and rotation of the spine and hips from such positions
as fixed prone lying and lax stoop stride standing.

Example: (i) *Neck rest fixed prone lying; Trunk bending backward with turning (Fig.* 101).

(ii) *Lax stoop back lean stride standing (heels* 12–15 *in.
in front of upright); Trunk stretching 'vertebra
by vertebra' in different planes (Fig.* 102).

Strengthening Exercises

(Flexors and Rotators)

Elementary.—
Grade 1.
1. Stride lying; Trunk turning with Head bending forward
and single Arm carrying across the chest.

Grade 2.
1. Stride lying; upper Trunk bending forward with turning
and single Arm carrying across the chest. (*See Fig.* 98, p. 71.)

Intermediate.—
Grade 1.
1. No progression.

2. Fixed lying; Trunk bending forward with turning, with
assistance from arms.

Grade 2.
1. No progression.

2. Fixed slight crook lying; Trunk bending forward with turning and single Arm carrying across the chest.

Advanced.—
Grade 1.
1. No progression.

2. Wing fixed crook lying; Trunk bending forward with turning. (*See Fig.* 99, p. 71.)

Grade 2.
1. No progression.

2. Neck rest fixed crook lying; Trunk bending forward with
turning. (*Fig.* 99, p. 71.)

Strengthening Exercises

(Extensors and Rotators)

Elementary.—

Grade 1.

1. Fist bend lax stoop kneel sitting; Trunk stretching 'vertebra by vertebra' with turning. (*See Fig.* 100, p. 71.)

Grade 2.

1. As Exercise 1 above, but arms in neck rest.

2. Lax stoop back lean stride standing (heels 12–15 in. in front of upright); Trunk stretching 'vertebra by vertebra' in different planes. (*See Fig.* 102, p. 71.)

Intermediate.—

Grade 1.

1. Across bend lax stoop kneel sitting; Trunk stretching 'vertebra by vertebra' with turning and single Arm stretching and raising midway-upward.

2. As Exercise 2, Elementary, Grade 2, but arms in neck rest.

Grade 2.

1 and 2. No progressions.

3. Fixed prone lying; Trunk bending backward with turning.

Advanced.—

Grade 1.

1 and 2. No progressions.

3. Wing fixed prone lying; Trunk bending backward with turning.

Grade 2.

1 and 2. No progressions.

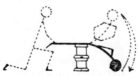

Fig. 103.

3. Neck rest fixed prone lying; Trunk bending backward with turning. (*See Fig.* 101, p. 71.)

4. Wing lax stoop fixed high thigh support across prone lying (balance benches, 2 high); Trunk stretching with turning to arch turn position (*Fig.* 103).

Grade 3.

1 and 2. No progressions.

3. Head rest fixed prone lying; Trunk bending backward with turning. (*See Fig.* 101, p. 71.)

4. As Exercise 4, Advanced, Grade 2, but arms in neck rest position.

CIRCUMDUCTORS OF THE SPINE

Types of Dynamic Exercises

The exercises are based on the following sequence of movement—Spine on Pelvis: Pelvis on Legs.

1. WORKING CIRCUMDUCTORS OF SPINE WITH HIP FLEXORS AND EXTENSORS.—Circumduction of the spine combined with flexion and extension of the hips from such starting positions as ride sitting and high ride sitting.

Example: *Wing ride sitting (balance bench: legs gripping bench sides); Trunk rolling (Fig.* 104).

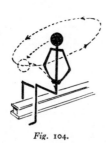 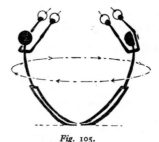

Fig. 104.   *Fig.* 105.

2. WORKING CIRCUMDUCTORS OF SPINE WITH HIP MUSCLES.— Circumduction of the spine combined with hip movements from stride standing and lax fall hanging (rings).

Example: (i) *Wing stride standing; Trunk rolling.*

       (ii) *Lax fall hanging (rings); rolling (Fig.* 105).

Mobilizing Exercises

Elementary.—

Grade 1.

1. Wing ride sitting (balance bench: legs gripping bench sides); Trunk rolling. (*See Fig.* 104, p. 74.)

2. Wing stride standing; Trunk rolling.

Grade 2.

1. Neck rest ride sitting (balance bench: legs gripping bench sides); Trunk rolling.

2. Neck rest stride standing; Trunk rolling.

Intermediate.—

Grade 1.

No progressions.

Grade 2.

1 and 2. No progressions.

3. Lax fall hanging (rings); rolling. (*See Fig.* 105, p. 74.)

Strengthening Exercises

See Trunk rolling exercises in previous section. The movements are performed more slowly than when used as mobility exercises.

CHAPTER VI

BREATHING EXERCISES

BREATHING exercises may be divided into four main groups:—

1. Bilateral exercises which are localized to the respiratory muscles. Such exercises consist of Apical, Costal, and Diaphragmatic breathing, and General deep breathing. The best starting positions for these exercises are crook half lying, half lying, and crook lying (*see* p. 80). The respiratory movements are localized by the use of the patient's hands, or with a webbing strap (p. 80).

Example: (i) *Crook half lying (hands on sides of lower ribs); lower lateral Costal breathing with light pressure from hands (Fig.* 106).

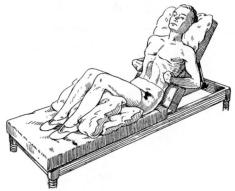

Fig. 106.—Lower lateral Costal breathing from crook half lying.

(ii) *Crook half lying (hand on upper abdomen); Diaphragmatic breathing, with emphasis on the contraction of the abdominal wall during expiration (Fig.* 107).

(iii) *Crook half lying (webbing strap round lower chest, with free ends held by hands); lower lateral Costal breathing with light pressure from strap (Fig.* 108).

Bilateral breathing exercises are used: (*a*) To increase the mobility of the thorax when the range of expiration or inspiration is reduced, (*b*) to ventilate the lungs and to prevent stagnation of mucous secretions, and (*c*) to teach correct breathing habits.

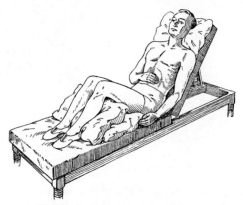

Fig. 107.—Diaphragmatic breathing.

2. Unilateral localized breathing exercises which are used in the treatment of certain chest conditions. For example, *Crook half lying (hand on side of left lower chest); left lower lateral Costal*

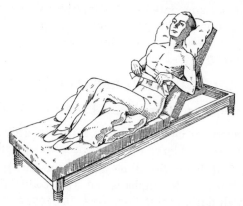

Fig. 108.—Using a strap to localize lower lateral Costal breathing.

breathing with hand pressure (Fig. 109), may be used in the treatment of empyema.

3. Arm exercises with breathing, e.g., *Stride sitting; Arm raising sideways-upward with breathing.*

4. Trunk exercises with breathing, e.g., *Stride sitting*; *Trunk bending sideways with breathing*.

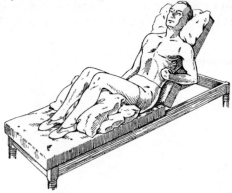

Fig. 109.—Unilateral Costal breathing.

Physiotherapists tend to concentrate on the first two groups of exercises, because in the remainder the associated arm and trunk movements neutralize the action of the respiratory muscles; hence there is no net gain in the respiratory function. For example, in the exercise *Arm raising sideways-upward with breathing* the ribs are fixed by the intercostal muscles, to stabilize the origin of the serratus anterior muscle; the fixation of the ribs neutralizes the upward dragging action of the pectoral muscles on the thorax, which would otherwise increase the range of inspiratory chest movements.

BILATERAL LOCALIZED BREATHING EXERCISES

Exercises to Increase the Expiratory Range

In these exercises emphasis is laid on prolonged, full expiration; inspiration must be as easy and shallow as possible.

1. Crook half lying (hand on upper abdomen); Diaphragmatic breathing, with emphasis on the contraction of the abdominal wall during expiration. (*See Fig.* 107, p. 77.)

2. Crook half lying (hands on sides of lower chest); lower lateral Costal breathing, with pressure by hands on ribs during expiration. (*See Fig.* 106, p. 76.)

3. Crook half lying (hands on sides of upper chest); upper lateral Costal breathing, with pressure by hands on ribs during expiration.

4. Crook half lying (fists on chest below clavicles); Apical breathing, with pressure by hands during expiration.

5. Crook half lying (hands on posterior surface of lower chest); posterior Basal breathing, with pressure by hands during expiration. (*Stoop sitting* is also used as a starting position for the exercise, especially when a strap is used to localize the chest movements.)

In Exercises 1–5 a webbing strap may be used to localize the chest movements. (See Fig. 108, p. 77.)

6. Crook half lying; general deep breathing, with emphasis on expiration.

7. Stride sitting; Trunk dropping loosely forward-downward to lax stoop position, with expiration, and Trunk stretching 'vertebra by vertebra' with shallow inspiration.

8. Stride sitting; Trunk turning with Arm swinging loosely at the sides: expiration during the backward turning movements, and shallow inspiration during the forward turning movements.

Exercises to Increase the Inspiratory Range

In these exercises emphasis is laid on deep inspiration, followed by ' normal ' expiration.

1. Crook half lying (hand on upper abdomen); Diaphragmatic breathing, with emphasis on the relaxation of the abdominal wall during inspiration. (*See Fig.* 107, p. 77.)

2. Crook half lying (hands on sides of lower chest); lower lateral Costal breathing with light pressure from hands. (*See Fig.* 106, p. 76.)

3. Crook half lying (hands on sides of upper chest); upper lateral Costal breathing with light pressure from hands.

4. Crook half lying (fists on chest below clavicles); Apical breathing with light pressure from hands.

In Exercises 1–4 a webbing strap may be used to localize the chest movements and to give light resistance. (See Fig. 108, p. 77.)

5. Crook half lying; general deep breathing.

6. Skipping and hopping exercises, running and swimming, to make the patient breathe deeply.

EXERCISES TO VENTILATE THE LUNGS AND PREVENT STAGNATION
OF MUCOUS SECRETIONS

The bilateral localized breathing exercises given in the previous lists are used, a full respiratory excursion being encouraged.

TECHNICAL POINTS

PRACTICAL TECHNIQUES

When the breathing exercises are first taught the instructor usually uses his hands to localize the movements for the patient. Later, when the patient understands the breathing techniques, he uses his hands or a webbing strap to localize the chest movements. (*See Figs.* 106–109, pp. 76–78.) Light resistance may be given with the hands or the strap when the exercises are used to increase the range of inspiration.

STARTING POSITIONS

Ideally, the breathing exercises are carried out from a starting position which gives the body the maximum support, and does not require any unnecessary muscle work, e.g., crook half lying (*Fig.* 106, p. 76), half lying, and crook lying (*Fig.* 110); whenever

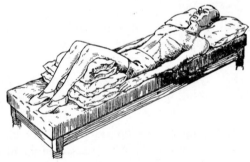

Fig. 110.—Crook lying as a starting position for localized breathing exercises: the thigh and head pillows ensure relaxation.

possible pillows are used to ensure complete relaxation. At a later date the instructor must make certain that the patient can perform the exercises correctly from other starting positions. These positions will depend on the clinical conditions for which breathing exercises are prescribed. For example, in the treatment of asthma the patient must be able to carry out certain breathing exercises when sitting and standing; in the early post-operative treatment of thoracoplasty the patient is required to control his breathing when sitting upright in bed.

Physical Education.—From the standpoint of physical education, sitting and standing may be used as starting positions for breathing exercises, in addition to crook lying, half lying, and crook half lying.

BREATHING EXERCISES IN PHYSICAL EDUCATION

Correct breathing habits are of considerable importance to the normal individual. For example, correct diaphragmatic breathing helps to prevent the development of lax abdominal muscles, and so indirectly assists in the maintenance of good posture. In the older age groups full diaphragmatic excursion is essential in order to ventilate the base of each lung adequately. Full ventilation prevents the accumulation of stagnant secretions in the base of the lung, which are prone to become infected. Infected secretions may contribute to the formation of such conditions as bronchiectasis and lung abscess.

CHAPTER VII

PELVIC-FLOOR EXERCISES

EXERCISES to strengthen the pelvic-floor muscles are used in the treatment of (1) Minor degrees of prolapse of the vaginal wall after childbirth, and (2) Stress incontinence caused by injury to the bladder sphincters, or, in women, by laxity of the muscles of the pelvic floor. Injury to the bladder sphincters may be produced by instrumentation or by prostatic resection.

Pelvic-floor exercises are also used in ante- and post-natal training.

TYPES OF PELVIC-FLOOR EXERCISES

The muscles of the pelvic floor are exercised indirectly in three ways:—

1. By contracting the hip adductors and the lower fibres of the gluteus maximus. This produces an associated contraction of the levator ani and the sphincters of the bladder.*

The hip adductors and extensors are exercised as separate groups or together from such starting positions as crook lying, lying, and standing. The muscles are also exercised in association with the sphincter ani.

Example: (i) *Crook lying (soft pillow between knees); Knee closing.*

(ii) *Crook lying (soft pillow between knees); Knee closing with Pelvis raising and contraction of Sphincter ani.*

2. By activating "the postural reflex between the abdominal wall and the pelvic floor whereby the pelvic floor contracts at the same time as the abdominal wall in order to withstand the strain of the increased intra-abdominal pressure".†

---

*† YATES-BELL, J. G., and COOKSEY, F. S. (1937), *J. chart. Soc. Massage med. Gymn.* (Congress number: Sept.), pp. 28, 31, and 32.

The abdominal wall is exercised either alone or in association with the gluteus maximus and external sphincter ani from such starting positions as crook lying and crook side lying.

Example: (i) *Crook lying (hand on upper abdomen); Diaphragmatic breathing with strong contraction of the Abdominal wall during expiration. (See Figs.* 107 and 110, pp. 77 and 80.)

(ii) *Crook lying (hand on upper abdomen); Diaphragmatic breathing with strong contraction of the Abdominal wall, plus Anal contraction, during expiration.*

(iii) *Crook lying; Pelvis tilting forward and backward, with emphasis on the backward tilting movement. (See Fig.* 111, which shows a different starting position.)

3. By contracting the external sphincter ani. It is possible that a contraction of this muscle is associated with a contraction of the pelvic-floor muscles.

The external sphincter ani may be exercised independently or in association with the gluteal, abdominal, and hip adductor muscles. Specific exercises for the sphincter are performed from such starting positions as lying, crook lying, and standing.

Example: *Crook lying; Anal contractions (attempting to draw anus up into pelvis).*

Pelvic-floor Exercises
Elementary.—
Grade 1.

1. Crook lying; Anal contractions (attempting to draw anus up into pelvis).

1A. As above, but with legs crossed. *Fig.* 111 shows the starting position.

2. Lying; Leg turning outward with Anal contractions.

3. Crook lying (soft pillow between knees); Knee closing.

4. Crook lying (hand on upper abdomen); Diaphragmatic breathing with strong contraction of the abdominal wall during expiration. (*See Figs.* 107 and 110, pp. 77 and 80.)

5. Crook lying; Pelvis tilting forward and backward, with emphasis on the backward tilting movement. (*See Fig.* 111, which shows a different starting position.)

5A. As Exercise 5, but taken from crook side lying.

5B. As Exercise 5, but taken from lying, with the legs crossed (*Fig.* 111).

Grade 2.

1 and 2. No progressions.

3. Crook lying (soft pillow between knees); Knee closing with Pelvis raising and Anal contractions (*Fig.* 112).

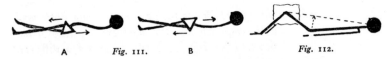

A   *Fig.* 111.   B   *Fig.* 112.

3A. Slight leg lift lying (legs crossed: heels supported on stool); Pelvis raising with Hip adduction.

3B. Inclined long sitting (ankles crossed); pressing Knees together with Gluteal and Anal contractions.

4. Crook lying (hand on upper abdomen); Diaphragmatic breathing with strong contraction of the abdominal wall, plus Anal contraction, during expiration.

5–5B. No progressions.

Intermediate.—
Grade 1.

1–3A. No progressions.

3B. Standing (legs crossed); Heel raising with Gluteal and Anal contraction.

4–5B. No progressions.

6. Walking while maintaining contraction of Gluteus maximus.

7. Standing; practising combined sustained Gluteal and Anal contraction.

8. Standing; practising coughing while maintaining combined sustained Gluteal and Anal contraction.

CHAPTER VIII

SHOULDER-GIRDLE EXERCISES

THESE exercises provide work for the muscles which activate the sternoclavicular and acromioclavicular joints *without* causing movement of the shoulder-joint. Examples of some dynamic exercises are given here.

ELEVATORS

Strengthening.—Sitting; Shoulder raising.
Mobilizing.—
1. Sitting; continuous Shoulder raising and lowering.
2. Sitting; alternate Shoulder shrugging.

DEPRESSORS

Strengthening.—
1. Sitting; Shoulder depression.
2. Lying; Shoulder depression.

ELEVATORS AND DEPRESSORS

Strengthening.—
1. Lying; Shoulder raising and depression, and return to starting position.
2. Sitting; Shoulder raising, lowering, depression, and return to starting position.

PROTRACTORS

Strengthening.—
1. Sitting; Shoulder rounding.
2. Lying; Shoulder rounding.

RETRACTORS

Strengthening.—
1. Sitting; Shoulder bracing.
2. Lying; Shoulder bracing.

4

PROTRACTORS AND RETRACTORS

Strengthening.—

1. Sitting; Shoulder rounding and bracing, and return to starting position.

2. Crook lying; exercise as above.

Mobilizing.—Sitting; Shoulder rounding and bracing.

ELEVATORS, PROTRACTORS, AND RETRACTORS

Mobilizing.—

1. Sitting; Shoulder-girdle rolling with emphasis on retraction.

2. As above, but with emphasis on protraction.

CHAPTER IX

COMBINED SHOULDER-JOINT
AND SHOULDER-GIRDLE EXERCISES

In the majority of the exercises given here the shoulder-girdle moves with the shoulder-joint; in certain of the exercises, however, shoulder-girdle movement is negligible, e.g., in rotation of the shoulder-joint from the neutral position.

1. SHOULDER FLEXORS AND FORWARD ELEVATORS OF ARM

Strengthening Exercises

Elementary.—

Grade 1.

1. Bend lying; single or double Elbow raising forward.

Grade 2.

1. Bend sitting; single or double Elbow raising forward or forward-upward.

2. Bend sitting; single or double Arm stretching forward-upward.

Grade 3.

1. Sitting; single or double Arm raising forward or forward-upward.

2. No progression.

Intermediate.—

Grade 1.

No progressions.

Grade 2.

1. Grasp walk forward standing (stick crosswise in front of body); Arm raising forward or forward-upward.*

---

* *Stick Exercises*: The types of sticks used for these exercises are broom-sticks and ash sticks. In general, broomsticks are more suitable for remedial work than ash sticks, because they are lighter.

2. Bend sitting (stick crosswise in front of chest); Arm stretching forward-upward.*

3. Grasp walk forward standing (stick crosswise in front of body); Arm bending, stretching forward-upward, and lowering to starting position.*

4. Reach grasp stoop stride standing (stick crosswise in front of body); Arm raising forward-upward.*

Advanced.—
Grade 1.

1. No progression.

2. First bend walk forward standing; single Arm punching forward or forward-upward.

3–4. No progressions.

5. Grasp walk forward standing (Indian clubs); single Arm swinging forward-upward, and club circling backward or forward *behind* the forearm to 3 counts.

5A. As above, but both arms are moved together (*Fig.* 113).

6. Grasp walk forward standing (Indian clubs); single Arm swinging forward-upward, and club circling backward or forward *in front* of the forearm to 3 counts.

6A. As above, but both arms are moved together.

Grade 2.

1–4. No progressions.

5–6A. Grasp walk forward standing (Indian clubs); Arm swinging forward-upward, and club circling (*a*) backward or forward *behind* the forearms to 2 counts, and (*b*) backward or forward *in front* of the forearms to 2 counts. (*See Fig.* 113.)

Mobilizing Exercises

Elementary.—
Grade 1.

1. Bend crook lying; alternate Elbow raising forward.

Grade 2.

1. Bend sitting; alternate Elbow raising forward.

Grade 3.

1. Crook lying; alternate Arm raising forward.

---

* *See* footnote, p. 87.

2. Toward standing (wall); single (affected) Arm 'crawling up the wall' (*Fig.* 114).

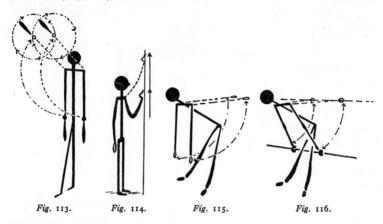

Fig. 113.   *Fig.* 114.   *Fig.* 115.   *Fig.* 116.

Intermediate.—

Grade 1.

1. Crook lying; alternate Arm swinging forward.

2. No progression.

3. Walk forward standing; alternate Arm swinging forward-upward.

4. Walk forward standing; Arm swinging forward-upward, with increasing range, to reach stretch position on the 4th count.

5. Walk forward standing; Arm swinging forward and forward-upward.

Grade 2.

1–2. No progressions.

3. Walk forward standing; alternate Arm swinging forward-upward with rhythmical pressing to 3 counts.

4. Grasp walk forward standing (stick crosswise in front of body); Arm swinging forward-upward with or without rhythmical pressing.*

5. Grasp walk forward standing (stick crosswise in front of body); Arm swinging forward and forward-upward.*

---

* *See* footnote, p. 87.

2. SHOULDER EXTENSORS

In these exercises movement of the shoulder-girdle occurs after the shoulder-joint has been extended fully. *See also* Exercises for the Depressors of the Arm, p. 94.

Strengthening Exercises

Elementary.—
Grade 1.
 1. Bend sitting; single or double Elbow raising backward.

Grade 2.
 1. Sitting; single or double Arm raising backward.

Intermediate.—
Grade 1.
 1. Prone lying; single or double Arm raising backward.
 2. Reach stoop stride standing; Arm raising backward (*Fig.* 115).

Grade 2.
 1. No progression.
 2. Reach grasp stoop stride standing (stick crosswise behind legs); Arm raising backward (*Fig.* 116).*

3. SHOULDER FLEXORS AND FORWARD ELEVATORS OF ARM WORKING WITH SHOULDER EXTENSORS

Many of the movements given in the previous sections may be combined (or the starting positions modified) to give wide range flexion and extension exercises of the shoulder-joint, with movement of the shoulder-girdle. Some examples are given below:—

 1. Walk forward standing; alternate Arm swinging forward-upward and downward-backward.

 2. Half crook side lying; single Arm swinging forward-upward and downward-backward.

 3. Reach stoop stride standing; Arm raising forward-upward, lowering, and raising backward as far as possible, and return to starting position.

---

* *See* footnote, p. 87.

4. SHOULDER ABDUCTORS AND SIDEWAYS ELEVATORS OF ARM

Strengthening Exercises

Elementary.—

Grade 1.

1. Sitting (affected upper limb resting on table, with shoulder abducted to about 90°, and elbow flexed); single Deltoid contractions.

Grade 2.

1. No progression.

2. Bend half lying; single or double Elbow raising sideways.

3. Half crook side lying; single Elbow raising sideways.

Grade 3.

1. No progression.

2. Bend sitting; single or double Elbow raising sideways.

3. Half crook side lying; single Arm raising sideways (*Fig.* 117, p. 93).

Grade 4.

1. No progression.

2. Half lying or sitting; single or double Arm raising sideways-upward.

3. No progression.

4. Bend sitting; single or double Arm stretching sideways-upward.

Intermediate.—

Grade 1.

No progressions.

Grade 2.

1–3. No progressions.

4. Bend grasp stride standing (stick crosswise in front of chest); Arm stretching sideways-upward.*

Advanced.—

Grade 1.

1–3. No progressions.

---

* *See* footnote, p. 87.

4. Fist bend stride standing; single Arm punching sideways or sideways-upward.

5. Grasp stride standing (Indian clubs); single Arm swinging sideways-upward, and club circling backward or forward *behind* the forearm to 3 counts.

5A. As No. 5, but both arms are moved together.

6. Grasp stride standing (Indian clubs); single Arm swinging sideways-upward, and club circling backward or forward *in front* of the forearm to 3 counts.

6A. As No. 6, but both arms are moved together.

Grade 2.

1–4. No progressions.

5–6A. Grasp stride standing (Indian clubs); Arm swinging sideways-upward, and club circling (*a*) backward *behind* the forearms to 2 counts, and (*b*) backward *in front* of the forearms to 2 counts.

Mobilizing Exercises

Elementary.—

Grade 1.

1. Bend half lying; alternate Elbow raising sideways.

Grade 2.

1. Bend sitting; alternate Elbow raising sideways.

2. Side toward standing (wall); single (affected) Arm 'crawling up the wall'. (*See Fig.* 114, p. 89, which shows the toward standing position.)

Grade 3.

1. Sitting; alternate Arm raising sideways-upward.

2. No progression.

Intermediate.—

Grade 1.

1. Stride standing; Arm swinging sideways-upward.

2. No progression.

3. Stride standing; Arm swinging to right and left, both arms moving in the same time and direction. (*See Fig.* 118, p. 93.)*

---

* This exercise provides some work for the shoulder adductors.

4. Low arm cross stride standing; Arm swinging sideways-upward.*

5. Stride standing; Arm swinging sideways-upward with increasing range to reach stretch position on the 4th count.

Grade 2.

1. Stride standing; Arm swinging sideways-upward to beat the fists together (1–2), and swinging downward-sideways to beat the sides of the thighs (3–4).*

2. No progression.

3. Wide grasp stride standing (stick crosswise in front of body); Arm swinging to right and left (*Fig.* 118).†

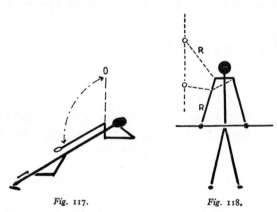

Fig. 117.   Fig. 118.

5. SHOULDER ADDUCTORS

In these exercises movement of the shoulder-girdle accompanies movement of the shoulder-joint. (*See also* Exercises for the Depressors of the Arm, p. 96.)

Strengthening Exercises

Elementary.—

Grade 1.

1. Sitting (hands clasped in front of body with elbows flexed to about 90°); pressing palms together strongly to produce static contractions of pectoralis major.

---

* This exercise provides some work for the shoulder adductors.
† *See* footnote, p. 87.

1A. Sitting (hands and forearms resting on thighs); single or double Arm pressing inward against the trunk to produce static contractions of pectoralis major.

Grade 2.

1 and 1A. No progressions.

2. Bend sitting; single Shoulder adduction, to move Elbow across the chest.

Grade 3.

1 and 1A. No progressions.

2. Sitting (elbows flexed to 90° and forearms in front of chest); single Shoulder adduction, to move Arm across the chest.

Grade 4.

1 and 1A. No progressions.

2. Stride standing; single or double Shoulder adduction, to move Arm(s) across the chest.

6. SHOULDER ABDUCTORS AND SIDEWAYS ELEVATORS OF ARM WORKING WITH SHOULDER ADDUCTORS

See Exercises marked with a star in Section 4, pp. 91–93. Certain of the movements given in Sections 4 and 5 may be combined to give wide-range abduction and adduction exercises of the shoulder-joint, with movement of the shoulder-girdle.

7. DEPRESSORS OF ARM AND SHOULDER EXTENSORS

Strengthening Exercises

Elementary.—

See Introductory Exercises to Arm bending from hanging, Circling on the rings or ropes, and Rope climbing, pp. 97–98.

Intermediate.—

Grade 1.

1. Under grasp standing (beam slightly above head level); Arm bending with take-off from floor.

Grade 2.

1. Under grasp hanging (beam); Arm bending (*Fig.* 119).
2. Inward grasp hanging (beam); Arm bending (*Fig.* 120).

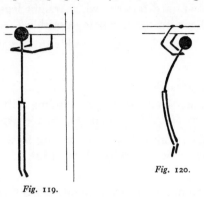

Fig. 119.

Fig. 120.

3. Heave grasp standing (rings or ropes); circling and return circling with bent knees, touching the floor with the feet at the end of the forward circling movement. (*See Fig.* 64 A, p. 52, for starting position, and *Fig.* 34, p. 37, for exercise with straight legs.)

4. Under grasp walk forward standing (beam at head height); circling forward-upward and downward-forward with bent knees. (*See Fig.* 65, p. 53, which shows the exercise performed with straight legs.)

Advanced.—

Grade 1.

1–2. No progressions.

3. Heave grasp standing (rings or ropes); circling and return circling with straight legs, touching the floor with the feet at the end of the forward circling movement. (*See Fig.* 64 A, p. 52, for starting position, and *Fig.* 34, p. 37, for movement.)

4. Under grasp walk forward standing (beam at head height); circling forward-upward and downward-forward with straight legs. (*See Fig.* 65, p. 53.)

5. Rope climbing: left or right Hand leading with Leg grasp.

Grade 2.

1–2. No progressions.

3. Stretch grasp standing (rings or ropes); circling and return circling with straight legs. (*See Fig.* 34, p. 37.)

4. Stretch under grasp standing (beam); circling forward-upward and downward-forward with straight legs. (*See Fig.* 65, p. 53, which shows an easier starting position.)

5. Rope climbing: Hand over Hand with Leg grasp.

Grade 3.

1–2. No progressions.

3. Inward grasp hanging (rings); circling and return circling with straight legs. (*See Fig.* 34, p. 37, for movement.)

4. Under grasp hanging (beam); circling forward-upward and downward-forward with straight legs. (*See Fig.* 65, p. 53, for movement.)

5. Rope climbing: Hand over Hand without Leg grasp.

8. DEPRESSORS OF ARM AND SHOULDER ADDUCTORS

Strengthening Exercises

Elementary.—
See Introductory Exercises to Arm bending from hanging, p. 97.

1. Stretch grasp high stoop standing (wall bars); Arm bending (*Fig.* 121).

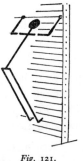

Fig. 121.

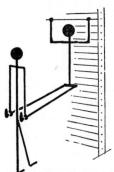

Fig. 122.

Intermediate.—
Grade 1.

1. Angle hanging (wall bars and living support); Arm bending (*Fig.* 122).

2. Over grasp standing (beam slightly above head level); Arm bending with take-off from floor.

Grade 2.

1. No progression.

2. Over grasp hanging (beam); Arm bending.

3. Over grasp hanging (beam); Arm walking sideways with Leg swinging from side to side. (*See Fig.* 83, p. 63.)

INTRODUCTORY EXERCISES

ARM BENDING FROM HANGING.—

Subject Working with Partner.—The partner takes some of the subject's body-weight during the arm bending. He stands behind him, and grasps him at the waist.

Exercise Performed from Standing.—The arm bending is performed from standing, with the beam arranged at stretch height. This allows the subject to rest his arms after each arm-bending movement.

CIRCLING ON RINGS OR ROPES.—

The subject attempts the circling in stages, first trying out a quarter turn, then a half circle, and finally a full circle. He need not attempt the return circle at first, but may let go of the rings or ropes and stand up when his feet touch the floor at the end of the forward circling.

Until the subject has acquired a good circling technique two supporters should stand on either side of him to give him confidence and, if necessary, to support him. It is also a wise precaution to put a mattress under the rings or ropes in case the subject accidentally loses his grasp.

CIRCLING ON THE BEAM.—

See p. 58.

ROPE CLIMBING.—

Leg Grip.—The subject practises taking and maintaining the leg grip, first with one foot behind the rope and then with the other. In the initial stages he sits on a stool which has been placed close to the rope. He grasps the rope as high as he can with both hands, and tries the leg grip without throwing any weight on to the arms. He must be taught to carry the feet well forward when he has gripped the rope, to prevent it from being held between the thighs instead of the knees; this would result in a weak grip.

The subject tests the grip by lifting his buttocks from the stool and swinging on the rope, or using his legs as in climbing. Thus he bends the arms and stretches the legs without losing his grip with the knees and feet, and then sits down on the stool again by allowing the arms to straighten out and the knees to bend.

Ascending and Descending the Rope.—When the leg grip has been mastered the subject practises ascending and descending the rope from standing, without raising the hands much higher than stretch height. He then progresses to the full climb.

9. SHOULDER PROTRACTORS

Protraction of the shoulder-joint "is a movement in which the fully abducted arm is brought towards the fully flexed position".* The movement is associated with protraction of the shoulder-girdle.

Strengthening Exercises

Elementary.—

Grade 1.

1. Neck rest lying; single or double Arm protraction.

Grade 2.

1. No progression.

Grade 3.

1. Yard (palms forward) lying; single or double Arm protraction (*Fig.* 123).

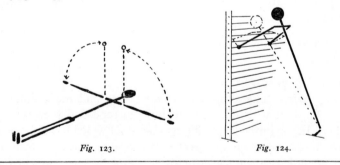

Fig. 123.   *Fig.* 124.

---

* APPLETON, A. B. (1946), *Surface and Radiological Anatomy*, 2nd ed., p. 46. Cambridge: Heffer & Sons.

Intermediate.—

Grade 1.

1. No progression.

2. Inclined prone falling (wall bars: hands between shoulder and hip height); Arm bending (*Fig.* 124).

Grade 2.

1. No progression.

2. Inclined prone falling (beam below hip height: hands supported); Arm bending. (*See Fig.* 25, p. 34.)

Advanced.—

Grade 1.

1. No progression.

2. Prone falling; Arm bending. (*See Fig.* 28, p. 36.)

Grade 2.

1. No progression.

2. Horizontal prone falling; Arm bending. (*See Fig.* 29, p. 36.)

10. SHOULDER RETRACTORS

Retraction of the shoulder-joint is a movement in which the fully flexed arm is moved backward through the horizontal plane to the fully abducted position. The movement is associated with retraction of the shoulder-girdle.

Strengthening Exercises

Elementary.—

Grade 1.

1. Neck rest (elbows forward) stoop stride standing; single or double Elbow parting.

Grade 2.

1. No progression.

Grade 3.

1. Reach stoop stride standing; single or double Arm parting.

Intermediate.—

Grade 1.

1. No progression.

2. Reach grasp stoop stride standing (stick crosswise in front of body); Arm bending to bring stick to chest (*Fig.* 125).*

3. Over grasp fall hanging (beam at shoulder height); Arm bending. (*See Fig.* 39, p. 42.)

Grade 2.

1–2. No progressions.

3. Over grasp fall hanging (beam below shoulder height); Arm bending.

Grade 3.

1–2. No progressions.

3. Over grasp horizontal fall hanging (beam and living support); Arm bending. (*See Fig.* 41, p. 43.)

11. SHOULDER PROTRACTORS AND RETRACTORS

For definition of protraction and retraction of the shoulder-joint *see* previous sections.

Strengthening Exercises

Elementary.—

Grade 1.

1. Neck rest (elbows forward) sitting; single or double Elbow parting.

Grade 2.

1. Reach sitting; single or double Arm parting.

Grade 3.

1. Yard (palms forward) sitting; Arm carrying forward to press the palms together strongly, followed by Arm carrying backward to the full extent, and return to starting position.

Intermediate.—

Grade 1.

1. Reach grasp walk forward standing (stick crosswise in front of chest); stick carrying backward to the right, and return to starting position, and repetition of movement to the left.*

2. Reach grasp walk forward standing (stick crosswise in front of chest); Arm bending in horizontal plane to bring stick to chest.*

---

* *See* footnote, p. 87.

Grade 2.

No progressions.

Advanced.—

Grade 1.

1–2. No progressions.

3. Under bend stride standing; single Arm punching horizontally across the chest (*Fig.* 126).

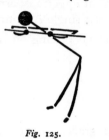
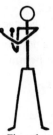

Fig. 125.   Fig. 126.

Mobilizing Exercises

Intermediate.—

Grade 1.

1. Reach grasp walk forward standing (stick crosswise in front of chest); stick swinging backward and forward in the horizontal plane.*

2. Across bend walk forward standing; Elbow pressing backward with Arm flinging on the 3rd count.

3. Yard (palms forward) walk forward standing; Cabman's swing.

12. LATERAL ROTATORS OF SHOULDER-JOINT

Strengthening Exercises

See Exercises in which the arms are raised sideways-upward, p. 91. In these exercises the lateral rotators of the shoulder-joint act with the shoulder-abductors and the elevators of the arm.

Elementary.—

Grade 1.

1. Forearm reach sitting; single or double Arm turning outward (*Fig.* 127).

---

* *See* footnote, p. 87.

2. Sitting; single or double Arm turning outward.

Grade 2.

1. Forward heave lying; single or double Arm turning inward through 90° (*Fig.* 128).

2. No progression.

Grade 3.

1. Half crook side lying (elbow of uppermost arm flexed to 90°, and forearm in contact with chest); single Arm turning outward.

2. Sitting; single or double Hand placing on back of neck or slight distance behind neck.

Intermediate.—
Grade 1.

1. No progression.

2. As Exercise 2, in previous grade, but performed in prone lying.

3. Heave grasp sitting (stick crosswise); Arm turning inward to bring stick against chest. *Fig.* 129 shows the exercise taken from walk forward standing.*

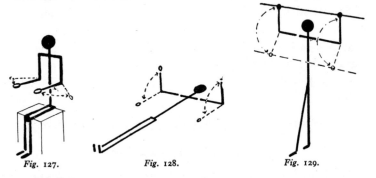

Fig. 127.   Fig. 128.   Fig. 129.

13. MEDIAL ROTATORS OF SHOULDER-JOINT

Strengthening Exercises

Elementary.—
Grade 1.

1. Forearm reach sitting; single or double Arm turning inward.

2. Sitting; Arm turning inward.

---

* *See* footnote, p. 87.

Grade 2.

1. Heave lying; single or double Arm turning inward through · 90° (*Fig.* 130).

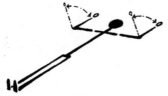

Fig. 130.

2. No progression.

Grade 3.

1. No progression.

2. Sitting; single or double Hand placing on lumbar spine or slight distance behind it.

Intermediate.—

Grade 1.

1. Heave grasp lying (stick crosswise); Arm turning inward through 90°.*

2. As Exercise 2, in previous grade, but performed in prone lying.

14. LATERAL AND MEDIAL ROTATORS OF SHOULDER-JOINT

Many of the movements given in the two previous sections may be combined to give wide-range rotation exercises of the shoulder-joint. Two examples of mobilizing exercises are given here:—

1. Forearm reach sitting; Arm turning outward and inward continuously to a given count.

2. Sitting; alternate Hand placing behind the neck and the lumbar spine.

15. SHOULDER CIRCUMDUCTORS AND ELEVATORS OF ARM

Mobilizing Exercises

Elementary.—

Grade 1.

1. Bend sitting; single or double Elbow circling forward or backward.

---

* *See* footnote, p. 87.

2. Bend sitting; alternate Elbow circling forward or backward.

Grade 2.

No progressions.

Grade 3.

1. Sitting or walk forward standing; single or double Arm circling forward or backward.

1A. Sitting or walk forward standing; alternate Arm circling forward or backward.

2. Stride standing; single Arm circling in the frontal plane, the circling starting in an outward or inward direction.

2A. As Exercise 2, but both arms are moved together and in the same direction.

Intermediate.—
Grade 1.

1. Walk forward standing; single or double Arm swinging in a circle: forward or backward.

1A. Walk forward standing; alternate Arm swinging in a circle: forward or backward.

1B. Forward fallout standing (hand on thigh); single Arm swinging in a circle: forward or backward (*Fig.* 131).

2. Stride standing; single Arm swinging in a circle in the frontal plane, the circling starting in an outward or inward direction.

2A. As Exercise 2, but the arms are moved together and in the same direction.

Grade 2.

1. Wide grasp walk forward standing (stick crosswise in front of body); Arm circling forward-upward (Arm bending to bring stick close to chest, stretching forward-upward to stretch position, and lowering downward-forward to starting position).*

1A–2. No progressions.

2A. Wide grasp stride standing (stick crosswise in front of body); Arm swinging in a circle in the frontal plane, the circling starting to the right or left.*

---

* *See* footnote, p. 87.

Advanced.—

Grade 1.

1. Grasp walk forward standing (Indian clubs); single or double Arm swinging in a forward or backward circle.

1A, B. No progressions.

2. Grasp stride standing (Indian clubs); single Arm swinging in a circle in the frontal plane, the circling starting in an outward or inward direction.

2A. As Exercise 2, but the arms are moved together and in the same direction (*Fig.* 132).

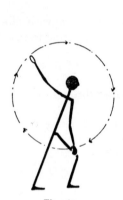 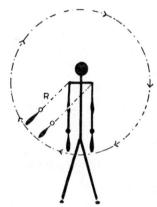

Fig. 131.   *Fig. 132.*

Grade 2.

1. Grasp walk forward standing (Indian clubs); single Arm swinging in a forward circle, pausing in the half high reach position to swing the club backward *behind* the forearm to 1 count.

1A, B. No progressions.

1C. As Exercise 1, but the arms are moved together.

2. Grasp stride standing (Indian clubs); single Arm swinging in a circle in the frontal plane, pausing in the half high yard position to circle the club backward *behind* the forearm to 1 count.

2A. As Exercise 2, but the arms are moved together.

Strengthening Exercises

See Exercises in previous section. The movements are performed more slowly than when used as mobility exercises.

Chapter X

ELBOW EXERCISES

FLEXORS

Strengthening Exercises

Elementary.—

Grade 1.

1. Sitting (forearms and hands resting on table, with elbows flexed and forearms supinated); single Biceps contractions.

Grade 2.

1. No progression.

2. Lying; single or double Elbow bending through 90°.

Grade 3.

1. No progression.

2. Sitting; single or double Elbow bending.

Intermediate.—

Grade 1.

1. No progression.

2. Grasp standing (stick crosswise in front of body); Arm bending.*

3. Reach grasp stoop stride standing (stick crosswise in front of body); Arm bending to bring stick to chest. (*See Fig.* 125, p. 101.)*

Grade 2.

1–3. No progressions.

4. Grasp stride standing (Indian clubs); single Arm swinging across the chest, bending (allowing the upper arm to return to side of trunk), and club circling backward *behind* the forearm to 3 counts, and stretching downward.

---

* *Stick Exercises* : The types of sticks used for these exercises are broomsticks and ash sticks. In general, broomsticks are more suitable for remedial work than ash sticks, because they are lighter.

4A. As previous exercise, but both arms are moved together.

5. Stretch grasp high stoop standing (wall bars); Arm bending. (*See Fig.* 121, p. 96.)

6. Over grasp fall hanging (beam at shoulder height); Arm bending. (*See Fig.* 39, p. 42.)

Advanced.—
Grade 1.

1–4A. No progressions.

5. Angle hanging (wall bars and living support); Arm bending. (*See Fig.* 122, p. 96.)

6. Over grasp fall hanging (beam below shoulder height); Arm bending.

7. Under grasp or over grasp hanging (beam slightly above head height); Arm bending with take-off from floor. (*See Fig.* 119, p. 95, and *Fig.* 133, of Arm bending without take-off.)

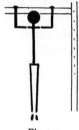

Fig. 133.

Grade 2.

1–5. No progressions.

6. Over grasp horizontal fall hanging (beam and living support); Arm bending. (*See Fig.* 41, p. 43.)

7. Under grasp or over grasp hanging (beam); Arm bending. *Fig.* 133 shows Arm bending from over grasp hanging. (*See also Fig.* 119, p. 95.)

EXTENSORS
Strengthening Exercises
Elementary.—
Grade 1.

1. Sitting; single Triceps contractions.

1A. Lying; single Arm pressing downward.

Grade 2.

1–1A. No progressions.

2. Bend lying; single or double Arm stretching forward.

Grade 3.

1–1A. No progressions.

2. Bend sitting; single or double Arm stretching sideways-upward.

Intermediate.—
Grade 1.

1–1A. No progressions.

2. Bend grasp sitting (stick crosswise); Arm stretching sideways-upward.*

Grade 2.

1–2. No progressions.

3. Grasp stride standing (Indian clubs); single Arm swinging in a circle in the frontal plane (the circling starting in an outward or inward direction), pausing in the half stretch position to (*a*) bend the arm, so that the hand is brought behind the head, and (*b*) circle the club backward *behind* the forearm to 3 counts.

4. Inclined prone falling (wall bars: hands between shoulder and hip height); Arm bending. (*See Fig.* 124, p. 98.)

Advanced.—
Grade 1.

1–3. No progressions.

4. Inclined prone falling (beam below hip height: hands supported); Arm bending. (*See Fig.* 25, p. 34.)

Grade 2.

1–3. No progressions.

4. Horizontal prone falling; Arm bending. (*See Fig.* 29, p. 36.)

FLEXORS AND EXTENSORS

Strengthening Exercises

Elementary.—
Grade 1.

1. Lying; single or double Elbow bending.

---

* *See* footnote, p. 106.

Grade 2.

1. Bend sitting; single or double Arm stretching forward.

1A. Bend sitting; Arm stretching forward and sideways.

Intermediate.—

No progressions.

Advanced.—

Grade 1.

1. Fist bend walk forward standing; single Arm punching forward, and strong return movement.

1A. Fist bend stride standing; single Arm punching sideways, and strong return movement.

Mobilizing Exercises

Elementary.—

Grade 2.

1. Sitting or walk forward standing; alternate Elbow bending and stretching, the extremes of both movements being emphasized.

2. As above, but elbow flexion is combined with supination of forearm, and elbow extension is combined with pronation of forearm.

Intermediate.—

Grade 1.

1. Walk forward standing; single Elbow bending and stretching, with gentle rhythmical pressing to 3 counts on reaching the extremes of movement.

2. No progression.

3. Wide grasp stride standing (stick crosswise in front of body); Arm circling forward-upward (Arm bending to bring stick to chest, stretching forward-upward to stretch position, and lowering downward-forward to starting position).*

---

* *See* footnote, p. 106.

Chapter XI

FOREARM, WRIST, AND HAND EXERCISES

THE weight of the moving part in these exercises is relatively small; hence it is impracticable to give lists of progressive exercises as in previous chapters. Specimen exercises for the individual muscle groups are listed.

I. FOREARM EXERCISES

PRONATORS

Strengthening Exercises

Elementary.—

1. Sitting (elbows flexed to 90°, with palms together and fingers pointing forward-downward); single or double Forearm pronation.

Intermediate.—

2. Half forearm reach grasp standing (stick vertical with distal end pointing downward: hand grasps shaft some distance from

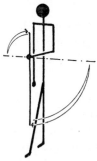

Fig. 134.

proximal end); single Forearm turning inward until stick is in horizontal position with distal end pointing outward. *Fig.* 134 shows the exercise taken from walk forward standing.*

---

* *Stick Exercises*: The types of sticks used for these exercises are broomsticks and ash sticks. In general, broomsticks are more suitable for remedial work than ash sticks, because they are lighter.

3. Starting position as above, but distal end of stick points upward; single Forearm turning outward until stick is in horizontal position with distal end pointing outward.*

Advanced.—

4. Stick exercises as above, but hand grasps the stick close to the proximal end.*

SUPINATORS

Strengthening Exercises

Elementary.—

1. Forearm reach sitting (palms downward, lax wrists and fingers); single or double Forearm supination, so that the fingers point upward. *Fig.* 127, p. 102, shows Forearm reach position.

Intermediate.—

2. Half forearm reach grasp standing (stick vertical with distal end pointing downward: hand grasps shaft some distance from proximal end); single Forearm turning outward until stick is in horizontal position with distal end pointing inward. *Fig.* 135 shows the exercise taken from walk forward standing.*

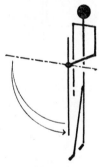

Fig. 135.

2A. Starting position as above, but distal end of stick points upward; single Forearm turning inward until stick is in horizontal position with distal end pointing inward.*

Advanced.—

3. Stick exercises as above, but the hand grasps the stick close to the proximal end.*

---

* *See* footnote, p. 110.

PRONATORS AND SUPINATORS

Strengthening Exercises

Elementary.—

1. Forearm reach sitting (lax fingers); single or double Forearm turning. *Fig.* 127, p. 102, shows Forearm reach position.

Intermediate.—

2. ' Screwing ' inward and outward movements with a stick against self-resistance (*Fig.* 136).*

3. Half forearm reach grasp standing (palm downward, and stick horizontal, with distal end pointing outward: hand grasps shaft some distance from proximal end); single Forearm turning outward until stick is in horizontal position with distal end pointing inward (*Fig.* 137).*

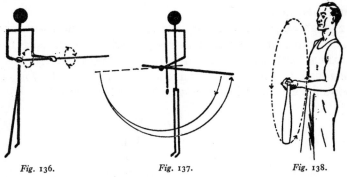

Fig. 136. Fig. 137. Fig. 138.

3A. Starting position as above, but palm faces upward; single Forearm turning inward until stick is in horizontal position with distal end pointing inward.*

Advanced.—

4. Stick exercises as above. In the ' screwing ' movements the self-resistance is increased, and in the Forearm turning exercises the hand grasps the stick close to the proximal end.

5. Grasp stride standing (Indian clubs); single Elbow bending to 90°, and club swinging in a circle in an outward or inward direction. *Fig.* 138 shows a swinging which starts in an outward direction.

5A. As Exercise 5, but both arms are used at the same time.

---

* *See* footnote, p. 110.

6. Grasp walk forward standing (Indian clubs); single Arm swinging forward-upward, and club circling (*a*) backward *behind* the forearm to 2 counts, and (*b*) backward *in front* of the forearm to 2 counts.

6A. As Exercise 6, but both arms are moved at the same time.

Mobilizing Exercises

Elementary.—

1. Forearm reach sitting (lax fingers); single, double, or alternate Forearm turning inward and outward.

Intermediate.—

2. Forearm reach sitting (lax fingers); single or double Forearm turning inward and outward with rhythmical pressing to a given count.

3. Forearm reach sitting (lax wrists and fingers); alternate Forearm turning inward and outward with a shaking motion.

4. Sitting or walk forward standing; alternate Elbow bending (with Forearm supination) and stretching (with Forearm pronation).

5. Half forearm reach grasp standing (stick in vertical position, and grasped at centre of shaft); single Forearm turning inward and outward with a swinging motion.

6. ' Screwing ' inward and outward movements with a stick. (*See Fig.* 136, p. 112.)

Advanced.—

See Club Exercises in previous section.

II. WRIST EXERCISES

The muscles of the wrist are exercised synergically when the fingers are used, e.g., in gripping, the wrist extensors act synergically. Exercises and simple occupations for the fingers should always be used in association with specific wrist exercises.

WRIST FLEXORS

Strengthening Exercises

Elementary.—

1. Forearm reach sitting (palms upward, lax fingers); single or double Wrist flexion (*Fig.* 139).

2. As above, but with Finger flexion.

Intermediate.—

3. Half grasp standing (palm forward, and stick held obliquely forward with distal end resting on floor: hand grasps shaft some distance from proximal end); single Wrist bending (*Fig.* 140).*

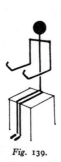
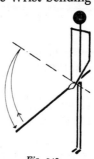

Fig. 139.   *Fig.* 140.

4. Forearm reach grasp standing (palms upward: stick crosswise); Wrist flexion. *Fig.* 127, p. 102, shows Forearm reach position.*

Advanced.—

5. As Exercise 3, but the hand grasps the stick close to the proximal end.*

WRIST EXTENSORS
Strengthening Exercises

Elementary.—

1. Forearm reach sitting (palms downward, lax fingers and wrists); single or double Wrist extension. *Fig.* 127, p. 102, shows Forearm reach position.

2. As Exercise 1, but with Finger extension.

Intermediate.—

3. Half grasp standing (palm backward, and stick held obliquely forward with distal end resting on floor: hand grasps shaft some distance from proximal end); single Wrist extension (*Fig.* 141).*

4. Forearm reach grasp standing (palms downward: stick crosswise); Wrist extension. *Fig.* 127, p. 102, shows Forearm reach position.*

---

* *See* footnote, p. 110.

Advanced.—

5. As Exercise 3, but the hand grasps the stick close to the proximal end.*

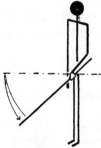

Fig. 141.

WRIST FLEXORS AND EXTENSORS

Strengthening Exercises

Elementary.—

1. Sitting (forearms and hands supported on table, palms facing inward and fingers lax); single or double Wrist flexion and extension, and return to starting position.

2. As above, but performed from Forearm reach sitting.

Mobilizing Exercises

Elementary.—

1. Forearm reach sitting (lax fingers); alternate Wrist flexion and extension (*Fig.* 142).

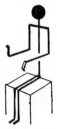

Fig. 142.

Intermediate.—

2. Forearm reach sitting (lax fingers); single Wrist flexion and extension, with gentle rhythmical pressing to a given count on reaching the extremes of movement.

---

* *See* footnote, p. 110.

3. Forearm reach sitting or standing (palms downward, lax fingers and wrists); alternate Wrist flexion and extension with a shaking motion (*Fig.* 142).

4. Standing or sitting (fingers interlocked, with elbows flexed and arms to sides); alternate Wrist flexion and extension.

WRIST ABDUCTORS

Strengthening Exercises

Elementary.—
1. Sitting (hands and forearms supported on table, palms facing inwards and fingers lax); single or double Wrist abduction.

2. As above, but with fingers straight.

Intermediate.—
3. Half grasp standing (palm inward, and stick held obliquely forward with distal end resting on floor: hand grasps shaft some distance from proximal end); single Wrist abduction. (*See Fig.* 141, p. 115.)*

Advanced.—
4. As Exercise 3, but the hand grasps the stick close to the proximal end.*

WRIST ADDUCTORS

Strengthening Exercises

Elementary.—
1. Sitting (forearms and hands resting on table, palms facing inwards, fingers lax); single or double Wrist adduction.

2. As above, but the fingers are kept straight.

WRIST ABDUCTORS AND ADDUCTORS

Mobilizing Exercises

Elementary.—
1. Sitting (forearms and hands resting on table, palms downward and fingers lax); alternate Wrist abduction and adduction.

2. As Exercise 1, but the fingers are kept straight.

---

* *See* footnote, p. 110.

Intermediate.—

3. As previous exercises, but with gentle rhythmical pressing to a given count on reaching the extremes of movement.

WRIST CIRCUMDUCTORS

Mobilizing Exercises

Elementary.—

1. Forearm reach sitting (lax fingers); single or double Wrist circling. *Fig.* 127, p. 102, shows Forearm reach position.

Advanced.—

2. Grasp stride standing (Indian clubs); single Elbow bending to 90°, and club swinging in a circle in an outward or inward direction. (*See Fig.* 138, p. 112.)

2A. As above, but both arms are used together.

3. Grasp walk forward standing (Indian clubs); single Arm swinging forward, and club circling (*a*) backward *behind* the forearm to 2 counts, and (*b*) backward *in front* of the forearm to 2 counts.

3A. As above, but both arms are moved together.

Strengthening Exercises

Advanced.—

See Club Exercises, above.

III. HAND EXERCISES

Simple occupations and everyday activities for the hand should always be used in association with specific exercises for the fingers and thumb.

EXERCISES TO STRENGTHEN THE GRIP

Elementary.—

1. Forearm reach sitting (lax fingers); strong Finger and Thumb bending, and slow recoil: each hand in turn or both hands together. *Fig.* 127, p. 102, shows Forearm reach position.

2. Sitting; squeezing a sorbo-rubber ball.

5

3. Sitting (corner of sheet of newspaper held in hand); rolling up paper into a tight ball in the palm of the hand without assistance from the free hand.

4. Sitting (end of unrolled crêpe bandage held in hand); rolling up bandage into a ball in the palm of the hand without assistance from the free hand.

Intermediate.—

5. Standing; stick travelling upward and downward, the hands changing places alternately (*Fig.* 143).*

6. As Exercise 5, but the stick is held in one hand, and the grasp is loosened and tightened alternately during the "travelling".*

7. Standing; stick throwing from hand to hand (*Fig.* 144).*

8. Reach grasp standing (stick crosswise); releasing stick and "dropping" the arms to catch it in the hands again.*

9. Bend grasp standing (stick crosswise); stick throwing upward and catching.*

10. Reach standing (palms downward: stick rests crosswise on arms); Arm lowering and stick catching (*Fig.* 145).*

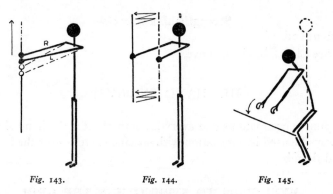

Fig. 143.　　　　Fig. 144.　　　　Fig. 145.

11. Inward grasp fall hanging (2 ropes); Arm bending. (*See Fig.* 39, p. 42, where a beam is shown in place of ropes.)

12. Stretch grasp standing (1 or 2 ropes); Arm bending with Ankle stretching to take weight off feet.

---

* *See* footnote, p. 110.

Advanced.—

13. Inward grasp horizontal fall hanging (2 ropes and living support); Arm bending. (*See Fig.* 41, p. 43, where a beam is shown in place of ropes.)

14. Over or under grasp hanging (beam); Arm bending. (*See Figs.* 133 and 119, pp. 107 and 95.)

15. Heave grasp walk forward standing (rings or ropes); circling and return circling with bent knees, touching the floor with the feet at the end of the forward circling movement. (*See Fig.* 34, p. 37, which shows a progression on the exercise.)

16. Rope climbing with Leg grasp.

EXERCISES TO STRENGTHEN THE FINGER AND THUMB EXTENSORS

Elementary.—

1. Sitting (forearms and hands resting on table, palms downward); Finger and Thumb extension: each hand in turn, or both hands together.

2. Forearm reach sitting (lax fingers); exercise as above.

EXERCISES TO INCREASE THE RANGE OF FINGER FLEXION OR EXTENSION

See Exercises given in two previous groups. Other exercises consist of: (*a*) Finger flexion or extension with rhythmical pressing to a given count, and (*b*) Wide range flexion and extension of the fingers and thumb.

Example: (i) *Half forearm reach (lax fingers); Finger flexion with rhythmical pressing to 3 counts. Fig.* 127, p. 102, shows Forearm reach position.

(ii) *Forearm reach sitting; Finger and Thumb bending and stretching: each hand in turn, or both hands together.*

EXERCISES TO STRENGTHEN THE INTRINSIC MUSCLES

Elementary.—

1. Sitting (forearms and hands resting on table, palms downward); single or double Hand shortening (flexion of the

metacarpophalangeal joints with the interphalangeal joints kept extended).

2. Starting position as above; Finger or Thumb parting, closing, and relaxation: each hand in turn, or both hands together.

3. Sitting (palms of hands together in front of chest, with fingers pointing upward and thumbs extended); Hand shortening (pressing finger tips together with flexion of the metacarpo-phalangeal joints—the interphalangeal joints being kept extended —and opposition of carpo-metacarpal joints).

EXERCISES TO STRENGTHEN THE THENAR AND HYPOTHENAR MUSCLES

See Exercises to Strengthen the Grip, pp. 117–119. Examples of some localized exercises of an elementary grade are given below:—

1. Forearm reach sitting (lax fingers); 'making O's' (touching the tip of each finger in turn with the tip of the thumb): each hand in turn, or both hands together. *Fig.* 127, p. 102, shows Forearm reach position.

2. Forearm reach sitting (palms upward, lax fingers); Palm hollowing (opposition of Thumb and 5th Finger): each hand in turn, or both hands together.

3. Forearm reach sitting; single or double Thumb circling slowly.

4. Forearm reach sitting (palms upward); single or double Thumb abduction and adduction.

Chapter XII

HIP EXERCISES

CERTAIN hip exercises in which the lower limbs are moved on the trunk are associated with movements of the pelvis and lumbar spine. These associated hip and trunk movements are described in the chapter on trunk exercises (pp. 32–75).

When leg exercises are used to activate the hip muscles the lower limbs ought not to be moved together as, for example, in *Leg raising* from lying. 'Double leg' exercises have a greater specific effect on the spinal muscles.

HIP FLEXORS

Strengthening Exercises

(*See also* Exercises for the Flexors of the Spine, pp. 32–40.)

Elementary.—
Grade 1.
   1. Lying; single Knee raising. (*See* p. 32.)

Grade 2.
   1. Lying; single high Knee raising. (*See Fig.* 22, p. 33.)

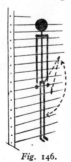

Fig. 146.

Intermediate.—
Grade 1.
   1. Low grasp back toward standing (wall bars); single high Knee raising (*Fig.* 146).

2. Lying; single Leg raising to 45°.

2A. Lying; single Leg raising.

3. Lying; single high Knee raising, Leg stretching forward to 45°, and lowering.

Grade 2.

1. No progression.

2. Low grasp back toward standing (wall bars); single Leg raising to 45°.

2A. As above, but single Leg raising.

Mobilizing Exercises

Elementary.—

1. Lying; alternate Knee raising.

2. Lying; alternate high Knee raising.

Intermediate.—

1. No progression.

2. Lying; cycling.

HIP EXTENSORS

Strengthening Exercises

(*See also* Exercises for the Extensors of the Spine, pp. 40–50. Hopping and Skipping Exercises may also be included.)

Elementary.—

Grade 1.

1. Lying or prone lying; single or double Gluteal contractions.

2. Lying; single Leg pressing downward.

Grade 2.

1–2. No progressions.

3. Reach grasp standing (wall bars or chair back); single Leg raising backward.

Intermediate.—

Grade 1.

1–2. No progressions.

3. Forehead rest prone lying; single Leg raising backward.

4. Low reach grasp standing (wall bars); Heel raising and Knee bending. (*See Fig.* 156, p. 132.)

5. Low reach grasp high standing (wall bars and balance bench); stepping down backward, sound Leg leading (1–2), and stepping up forward, sound Leg leading (3–4). (*See Fig.* 157, p. 132.)

6. Climbing the wall bars, 1–2 bars at a step.

Grade 2.

1–2. No progressions.

3. Prone kneeling; single Leg stretching and raising backward. (*See* leg movement of *Fig.* 61 B, p. 52.)

4. Half wing half low yard grasp standing (wall bars); Heel raising and Knee bending (*Fig.* 147).

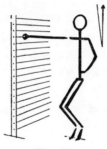

Fig. 147.

5. Reach grasp standing (wall bars and balance bench); stepping up forward, affected Leg leading (1–2), and stepping down backward, affected Leg leading (3–4).

6. Climbing the wall bars, 2–3 bars at a step.

7. Low reach grasp instep support standing (wall bars and stool); single Heel raising and Knee bending. (*See Fig.* 150, p. 124, which shows a progression on the exercise.)

8. Low reach grasp standing (wall bars); Heel raising and Knee full bending.

Advanced.—
Grade 1.

1–3. No progressions.

4. Wing standing; Heel raising and Knee bending.

5. Toward standing (balance bench or stool); stepping up forward, affected Leg leading (1-2), and stepping down backward, affected Leg leading (3-4).

6. No progression.

7. Half wing half low yard grasp instep support standing (wall bars and stool); single Heel raising and Knee bending. (*See Fig.* 147 for position of arms, and *Fig.* 150 for movement.)

8. Half wing half low yard grasp standing (wall bars); Heel raising and Knee full bending.

9. Low reach grasp high half standing (wall bars and plinth); single Knee full bending (*Fig.* 148).

Grade 2.

1-3. No progressions.

4. Neck rest standing; Heel raising and Knee bending.

5. Back toward standing (balance bench or stool); stepping up backward, affected Leg leading (1-2), and stepping down forward, affected Leg leading (3-4) (*Fig.* 149).

6. No progression.

7. Wing instep support standing (stool); single Heel raising and Knee bending (*Fig.* 150).

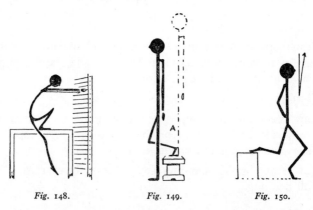

Fig. 148.   Fig. 149.   Fig. 150.

8. Wing standing; Heel raising and Knee full bending.

9. Half low yard grasp high half standing (wall bars and plinth); single Knee full bending.

Grade 3.

   1–3. No progressions.

   4. Stretch standing; Heel raising and Knee bending.

   5–6. No progressions.

   7. Stretch instep support standing (stool); single Heel raising and Knee bending.

   8. Neck rest standing; Heel raising and Knee full bending.

   9. Lax reach high half standing (plinth or high bench); single Knee full bending. (*See Fig.* 162, p. 134.)

Mobilizing Exercises

Intermediate.—

Grade 1.

   1. Forehead rest prone lying; single Leg raising backward with rhythmical pressing to 3 counts.

   2. Bend grasp high standing (wall bars); Knee full bending and stretching with Hand travelling down and up the bars. (*See Fig.* 168, p. 137.)

Grade 2.

   1. Prone kneeling; single Leg stretching and raising backward, with rhythmical pressing to 3 counts. (*See* leg movement of *Fig.* 61 B, p. 52.)

   2. No progression.

HIP FLEXORS AND EXTENSORS

Strengthening Exercises

(*See also* Exercises for the Flexors and Extensors of the Spine, pp. 50–57.)

Elementary.—

Grade 1.

   1. Half crook side lying; single slight Leg raising sideways, and carrying forward and backward, and return to starting position.

Grade 2.

   1. Lying; single high Knee raising, and return to starting position, followed by Leg downpressing.

Intermediate.—
Grade 1.

1. Reach grasp standing (wall bars); single high Knee raising, Leg stretching and raising backward, and return to starting position.

2. Prone kneeling; single high Knee raising, Leg stretching and raising backward, and return to starting position.

Mobilizing Exercises

Elementary.—

1. Half crook side lying; single slight Leg raising sideways, and carrying forward and backward to a given count (*Fig.* 151).

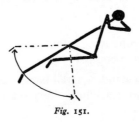

Fig. 151.

2. As above, but the Leg is swung forward and backward.

Intermediate.—

1. No progression.

2. Reach grasp high half standing (beam and block); single Leg swinging forward and backward.

HIP ABDUCTORS

Strengthening Exercises

(*See also* Exercises for the Lateral Flexors of the Spine, pp. 58–66.)

Elementary.—
Grade 1.

1. Reach grasp standing (wall bars); single Leg raising sideways.

2. Reach grasp standing (wall bars); single slight Knee raising (activates hip abductors of standing leg).

3. Hanging (wall bars or beam); Leg parting.

Grade 2.

1. Standing; single Leg raising sideways.

2. Standing; single Knee raising.

3. Half crook side lying; single Leg raising sideways.

HIP ADDUCTORS

Strengthening Exercises

(*See also* Exercises for the Lateral Flexors of the Spine, pp. 58–66.)

Elementary.—

Grade 1.

1. Close lying; pressing Knees together.

2. Crook lying; Knee parting and closing to press the knees together.

Grade 2.

1. No progression.

2. Yard (palms backward) vertical leg lift lying; Leg parting (*Fig.* 152).

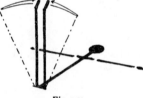

Fig. 152.

2A. Reverse hanging (wall bars); Leg parting. *Fig.* 86, p. 66, shows the reverse hanging position.

3. Hanging (wall bars or beam); Leg crossing.

4. Reach grasp high half standing (wall bars and block); single Leg crossing.

HIP ABDUCTORS AND ADDUCTORS

Strengthening Exercises

(*See also* Exercises for the Lateral Flexors of the Spine, pp. 58–66.)

Elementary.—
Grade 1.

1. Lying; single slight Leg raising, and carrying sideways and across the other leg, and return to starting position.

2. Lying; Leg parting and crossing, and return to starting position.

Grade 2.

1. Reach grasp standing (wall bars); single Leg raising sideways, lowering and crossing the standing leg, and return to starting position.

2. Hanging (wall bars or beam); Leg parting and crossing, and return to starting position.

Mobilizing Exercises

Elementary.—
Grade 1.

1. Lying; single slight Leg raising, and carrying sideways and across the other leg to a given count.

Grade 2.

1. As above, but the Leg is swung from side to side.

Intermediate.—
Grade 1.

1. Reach grasp high half standing (beam and block); single Leg swinging from side to side.

LATERAL ROTATORS OF HIP

Strengthening Exercises

Elementary.—
Grade 1.

1. Half crook side lying; single Leg turning outward.

2. Crook side lying; single Knee raising sideways, with feet kept together.

Grade 2.

1–2. No progressions.

3. High sitting (plinth); single Thigh turning outward, so that foot crosses other leg.

3A. As above, but both Thighs are turned outward (*Fig.* 153).

4. Prone lying (knees flexed to 90°); allowing Thighs to turn inward, so that feet are parted (*Fig.* 154).

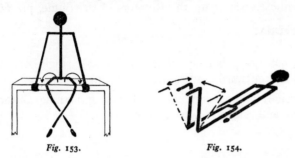

Fig. 153.   Fig. 154.

5. Reach grasp standing (wall bars); Hip turning outward, feet remaining in starting position.

MEDIAL ROTATORS OF HIP

Strengthening Exercises

Elementary.—
Grade 1.

   1. Lying (lax legs); Leg turning inward.

   2. Crook lying; Knee parting.

Grade 2.

   1–2. No progressions.

   3. High sitting (plinth); single Thigh turning inward, so that lower leg moves outward.

   3A. As above, but both Thighs are turned inward.

Fig. 155.

4. Stride prone lying (knees flexed to 90°); allowing Thighs to turn outward, so that ankles cross each other (*Fig.* 155).

LATERAL AND MEDIAL ROTATORS OF HIP

Strengthening Exercises

(*See also* Exercises for the Rotators of the Spine, pp. 66–70.)

Elementary.—
Grade 1.

1. Reach grasp half standing (wall bars); single Leg turning inward and outward, and return to starting position.

2. Stride lying; single or double Leg turning inward and outward, and return to starting position.

Grade 2.

1–2. No progressions.

3. High sitting (plinth); single or double Thigh turning inward and outward to the full extent, and return to starting position.

4. Prone lying; exercise as above.

5. Half crook lying; single Knee lowering sideways, raising to cross other leg, and return to starting position.

Mobilizing Exercises

As strengthening exercises, above, but the movements are performed in a continuous manner, e.g., *Stride lying; single Leg turning inward and outward continuously to a given count.* (*See also* Exercises for the Rotators of the Spine, pp. 66–70.)

CIRCUMDUCTORS OF HIP

Mobilizing Exercises

Elementary.—

1. Reach grasp high half standing (beam and block); single Leg circling or swinging in a circle.

2. Lying; single Leg circling.

3. Half crook side lying; single Leg circling.

Strengthening Exercises

See Exercises in previous section. The movements are performed more slowly than when used as mobility exercises. *See also* Exercises for the Circumductors of the Spine, p. 74.

CHAPTER XIII

KNEE EXERCISES

KNEE FLEXORS

Strengthening Exercises

(*See also* single Leg raising backward exercises, p. 122.)

Elementary.—
Grade 1.

1. Crook lying or sitting; single or double Hamstring contractions.

Grade 2.

1. No progression.

2. Forehead rest prone lying; single or double Knee bending to 90°.

Grade 3.

1. No progression.

2. High sitting (table or bench); single or double Knee bending.

3. Reach grasp standing (wall bars); single Knee bending backward.

KNEE EXTENSORS

Strengthening Exercises

(Hopping and Skipping Exercises may also be included.)

Elementary.—
Grade 1.

1. Long sitting or half lying; single or double Quadriceps contractions.

2. As Exercise 1, with Ankle or Foot movements, e.g., single Quadriceps contractions with Ankle bending.

Grade 2.

    1. Lying; single Leg raising to 45° with Knee firmly braced.

    1A. As above, but with Ankle bending.

    2. Lying ; single Leg raising with Knee firmly braced.

    2A. As above, but with Ankle bending.

    3. High sitting (plinth) ; single or double Knee stretching.

    3A. As above, but with Ankle bending.

Intermediate.—
Grade 1.

    1. Lying; single high Knee raising, Leg stretching forward to 45°, and slow lowering.

    1A–2A. No progressions.

    3. Low reach grasp standing (wall bars); Heel raising and Knee bending (*Fig.* 156).

    4. Low reach grasp high standing (wall bars and balance bench); stepping down backward, sound Leg leading (1–2), and stepping up forward, sound Leg leading (3–4) (*Fig.* 157).

    5. Climbing the wall bars, 1–2 bars at a step.

Grade 2.

    1–2A. No progressions.

    3. Half wing half low yard grasp standing (wall bars); Heel raising and Knee bending.

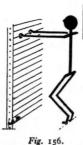 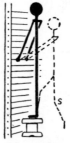 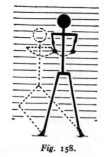

Fig. 156.   Fig. 157.   Fig. 158.

    4. Reach grasp standing (wall bars and balance bench); stepping up forward, affected Leg leading (1–2), and stepping down backward, affected Leg leading (3–4).

5. Climbing the wall bars, 2–3 bars at a time.

6. Low reach grasp standing (wall bars); Heel raising and Knee full bending.

7. Low reach grasp stride standing (wall bars); Heel raising and single Knee bending (*Fig.* 158).

8. Low reach grasp instep support standing (wall bars and stool); single Heel raising and Knee bending.

9. Short forward fallout standing; vigorous thrusting backward (*Fig.* 159).

Advanced.—
Grade 1.

1–2A. No progressions.

3. Wing standing; Heel raising and Knee bending.

4. Toward standing (balance bench or stool); stepping up forward, affected Leg leading (1–2), and stepping down backward, affected Leg leading (3–4).

5. No progression.

6. Half wing half low yard grasp standing (wall bars); Heel raising and Knee full bending.

7. Half wing half low yard grasp stride standing (wall bars); Heel raising and single Knee bending.

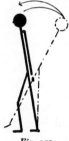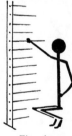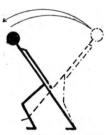

Fig. 159.   Fig. 160.   Fig. 161.

8. Half wing half low yard grasp instep support standing (wall bars and stool); single Heel raising and Knee bending (*Fig.* 160).

8A. Low reach grasp high half standing (wall bars and plinth); single Knee full bending. (*See Fig.* 148, p. 124.)

9. Forward fallout standing; vigorous thrusting backward (*Fig.* 161).

Grade 2.

1–2A. No progressions.

3. Neck rest standing; Heel raising and Knee bending.

4. Back toward standing (balance bench or stool); stepping up backward, affected Leg leading (1–2), and stepping down forward, affected Leg leading (3–4). (*See Fig.* 149, p. 124.)

5. No progression.

6. Wing standing; Heel raising and Knee full bending.

7. Wing stride standing; Heel raising and single Knee bending.

8. Wing instep support standing (stool); single Heel raising and Knee bending. (*See Fig.* 150, p. 124.)

8A. Half low yard grasp high half standing (wall bars and plinth); single Knee full bending.

9. No progression.

Grade 3.

1–2A. No progressions.

3. Stretch standing; Heel raising and Knee bending.

4–5. No progressions.

6. Neck rest standing; Heel raising and Knee full bending.

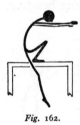

Fig. 162.

7. Neck rest stride standing; Heel raising and single Knee bending.

8. Neck rest instep support standing (stool); single Heel raising and Knee bending. *See Fig.* 150, p. 124, which shows the arms in wing position.

8A. Lax reach high half standing (plinth); single Knee full bending (*Fig.* 162).

9. No progression.

KNEE ROTATORS

Specific exercises for the knee rotators are not given here, because rotation of the knee is associated with flexion and extension movements. *See* Exercises for the Knee Flexors, p. 131, and Exercises for the Knee Extensors, pp. 131–134.

KNEE FLEXORS AND EXTENSORS

Strengthening Exercises

Knee flexion and extension movements may be combined in half crook side lying and high sitting, e.g., *High sitting (table or bench); single or double Knee bending, stretching, and return to starting position.* (*Fig.* 163.)

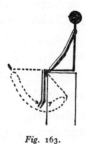

Fig. 163.

EXERCISES TO RESTORE THE RANGE OF KNEE FLEXION

a. **For use when the range of Knee flexion is less than 45°.**

1. Lying; affected Knee raising with heel in contact with supporting surface.

2. Half crook side lying; affected Knee bending and stretching continuously to a given count.

3. Prone lying; alternate Knee bending.

4. Prone lying; affected Knee bending with rhythmical pressing to a given count.

5. High sitting (plinth: heels resting on stool, with knees flexed); alternate Knee stretching.

b. **For use when the range of Knee flexion is between 45° and 90°.**

1. Lying; affected Knee raising with heel in contact with supporting surface.

2. Half crook side lying; affected Knee bending and stretching continuously to a given count.

3. Prone lying; alternate Knee bending.

4. Prone lying; affected Knee bending with rhythmical pressing to a given count.

5. High sitting (table or bench); alternate Knee stretching.

6. As above; alternate lower Leg swinging with Ankle bending and stretching (*Fig.* 164).

7. High sitting (table or bench); affected Knee attempted bending beyond stiff zone, and slow recoil.

8. Prone kneeling (knee position modified if necessary); Trunk moving backward and forward. (*See Fig.* 167, p. 137.)

8A. As Exercise 8, but with rhythmical pressing to a given count at end of backward movement.

9. Short walk forward standing (hands on forward knee); small range bending and stretching of forward knee (*Fig.* 165).

10. Low grasp inclined long sitting (balance bench); single high Knee raising, attempting to touch front edge of bench with heel (*Fig.* 166).

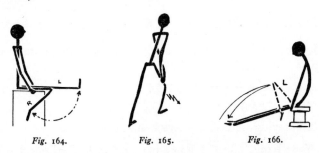

Fig. 164.   Fig. 165.   Fig. 166.

11. Bend grasp high standing (wall bars); Knee bending and stretching with Hand travelling down and up the bars. *See Fig.* 168, p. 137, which shows Hand travelling over two bars only.

c. **For use when the range of Knee flexion is over 90°.**

1–2. Omitted.

3. Prone lying; alternate Knee bending.

4. Prone lying; affected Knee bending with rhythmical pressing to a given count.

5. Omitted.

6. High sitting (table or bench); alternate lower Leg swinging forward and backward with Ankle bending and stretching. (*See Fig.* 164, p. 136.)

7. High sitting (table or bench); affected Knee bending as far as possible, and slow recoil.

8. Prone kneeling; Trunk moving backward and forward (*Fig.* 167).

8A. As above, but with rhythmical pressing to a given count at end of the backward movement.

9. Forward fallout standing (hands on forward knee); small range bending and stretching of forward knee. (*See Fig.* 165, p. 136.)

10. As Exercise 10, previous section

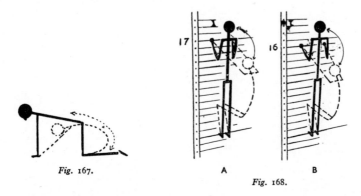

Fig. 167.

Fig. 168.

11. Bend grasp high standing (wall bars); Knee bending and stretching with Hand travelling down and up the bars. *Fig.* 168 shows Hand travelling over two bars only.

12. Lax stoop half kneeling (hands on floor); small range bending and stretching of forward knee (*Fig.* 169).

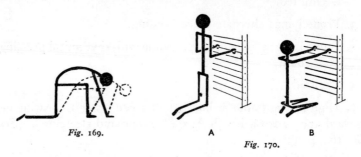

Fig. 169.   A

Fig. 170.   B

13. Forearm reach grasp kneeling (wall bars); attempting to assume kneel sitting (*Fig.* 170).

CHAPTER XIV

ANKLE AND FOOT EXERCISES

I. ANKLE EXERCISES

DORSIFLEXORS
Strengthening Exercises

(BALANCE exercises may also be included.)

Elementary.—
Grade 1.
   1. Half lying or long sitting (heels free); single or double Ankle bending with slight Knee raising.
   2. As above, but without Knee raising.

Grade 2.
   1. High sitting (plinth); single or double Ankle bending.
   2. No progression.
   3. Sitting; single or double Forefoot raising.

Intermediate.—
Grade 1.
   1. No progression.
   2. Reach grasp standing (wall bars); Forefoot raising.
   3. No progression.

PLANTAR-FLEXORS
Strengthening Exercises

(*See also* Exercises for the Knee Extensors, pp. 131–134. Hopping, Skipping, and Balance Exercises may also be included.)

Elementary.—
Grade 1.
   1. Half lying or long sitting; single or double Ankle stretching.

Grade 2.

   1. Prone lying (plinth: feet free); as previous exercise.

Grade 3.

   1. Sitting; single or double Heel raising.

Intermediate.—
Grade 1.

   1. Reach grasp standing (wall bars); Heel raising.

Grade 2.

   1. Half yard grasp standing (wall bars); Heel raising.

   2. Reach grasp instep support standing (wall bars and stool); single Heel raising. (*See Fig.* 171, which shows a progression on this exercise.)

Advanced.—
Grade 1.

   1. Wing standing; Heel raising.

   1A. Standing; Heel raising with Arm swinging forward and forward-upward.

   2. Half yard grasp instep support standing (wall bars and stool); single Heel raising.

   3. Walking on the toes with 'springing' steps.

Grade 2.

   1. Neck rest standing; Heel raising.

   1A. No progression.

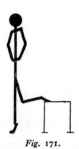

Fig. 171.

   2. Wing instep support standing (stool); single Heel raising (*Fig.* 171).

   2A. Lax yard half standing; single Heel raising.

   3. Running on the toes.

DORSIFLEXORS AND PLANTAR-FLEXORS

Strengthening Exercises

(Balance exercises may also be included.)

Many of the movements given in the two previous sections may be combined, e.g., *High sitting (plinth); Ankle bending, stretching, and return to starting position.*

Mobilizing Exercises

Elementary.—

1. Half lying or long sitting (heels free); alternate Ankle bending and stretching.

2. High sitting (plinth); as above.

3. Sitting (one ankle crossed over opposite knee); single Ankle bending and stretching continuously to a given count.

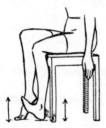

Fig. 172.

4. Sitting; alternate Forefoot and Heel raising (*Fig.* 172).

II. FOOT EXERCISES

INVERTORS

Strengthening Exercises

(Balance exercises may also be included.)

Elementary.—
Grade 1.

1. Half lying or long sitting (heels free); single or double Foot turning inward.

1A. As Exercise 1, with Toe flexion.

Grade 2.

1. High sitting (plinth); single or double Foot turning inward.

1A. As Exercise 1, with Toe flexion.

2. Sitting (one ankle crossed over opposite knee); single Foot turning inward.

3. Sitting; single or double inner Border raising.

4. Sitting; attempting to accentuate medial longitudinal arches.

Intermediate.—
Grade 1.

1–2. No progressions.

3. Reach grasp standing (wall bars) or standing; inner Border raising.

4. Starting position as Exercise 3; attempting to accentuate medial longitudinal arches.

EVERTORS

Strengthening Exercises

(Balance exercises may also be included.)

Elementary.—
Grade 1.

1. Half lying or long sitting (heels free); single or double Foot turning outward.

Grade 2.

1. High sitting (plinth); single or double Foot turning outward.

2. Sitting (one ankle crossed over opposite knee); single Foot turning outward.

3. Short stride sitting; single or double outer Border raising.

Intermediate.—
Grade 1.

1–2. No progressions.

3. Reach grasp short stride standing (wall bars) or standing; outer Border raising.

INVERTORS AND EVERTORS

Strengthening Exercises

(Balance exercises may also be included.)

Certain of the movements given in the two previous sections may be combined, e.g., *High sitting (plinth); Foot turning inward and outward, and return to starting position.*

Mobilizing Exercises

Elementary.—

1. Half lying or long sitting (heels free); alternate Foot turning inward and outward continuously to a given count.

2. High sitting (plinth); as above.

3. Sitting (one ankle crossed over opposite knee); single Foot turning inward and outward continuously to a given count.

4. Short stride sitting; inner and outer Border raising continuously to a given count.

CIRCUMDUCTORS

Mobilizing Exercises

Elementary.—

1. Half lying or long sitting (heels free); single or double Foot circling.

2. High sitting (plinth); as above.

3. Sitting (one ankle crossed over opposite knee); single Foot circling.

N.B.—Emphasis may be placed on a particular part of the circling, e.g., Circling with emphasis on inversion.

Strengthening Exercises

The movements given in the previous section may also be used as strengthening exercises; they are then performed more slowly.

INTRINSIC MUSCLES

Strengthening Exercises

Elementary.—

1. Sitting; single or double Foot shortening (flexion of the metatarsophalangeal joints, with extension of the interphalangeal joints) (*Fig.* 173).

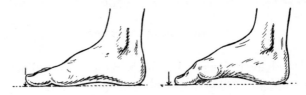

Fig. 173.—Foot shortening: an exercise for the intrinsic muscles.

1A. Half lying or long sitting (feet supported by footboard, with ankles dorsiflexed); single or double Foot shortening. *See above.* (*Fig.* 174.)

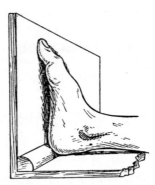

Fig. 174.—Foot shortening adapted for bed use: the feet are supported by a footboard.

2. Half lying or long sitting; Toe parting and closing.

2A. Sitting (feet resting on floor or in tray of sand); Toe parting and closing.

3. Sitting (toes resting on book); Toe flexion at the metatarsophalangeal joints, with extension of the interphalangeal joints: each foot in turn, or both together (*Fig.* 175).

4. Sitting (feet resting on book, with all the toes free); Toe flexion at the metatarsophalangeal joints, with extension of the interphalangeal joints: each foot in turn, or both together.

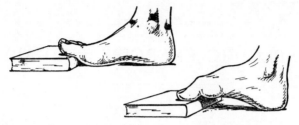

Fig. 175.—Another exercise for the intrinsic muscles.

Intermediate.—

1. Standing; single or double Foot shortening. (*See* Exercise 1, Elementary grade.)

2. No progression.

3. Standing; practising correct 'push off' movement from toes in walking (interphalangeal joints of toes must be kept extended).

TOE FLEXORS AND EXTENSORS

The strengthening exercises for the flexors and extensors of the toes consist of strong flexion and extension movements, followed by a slow return to the starting position.

Example: *Half lying or long sitting; strong Toe bending, and slow recoil: each foot in turn, or both together.*

The mobilizing exercises consist of flexion and extension movements which are performed in a continuous manner.

Example: *Long sitting; Toe bending and stretching continuously to a given count: both feet together.*

PART III

SPECIFIC EXERCISE THERAPY

CHAPTER XV

CONSTRUCTION AND USE OF TABLES
OF SPECIFIC EXERCISES

THE tables consist of lists of movements which provide exercise
for a particular area of the body; they are used in the treatment of
localized lesions, such as fractures, chest diseases, and post-
operative abdominal conditions. A series of graded tables is
required to provide smooth, progressive exercise from the early
to the late phase of recovery. If a patient's condition remains
stationary for a considerable time, the exercises are changed or
modified to maintain interest.

The patients are treated individually, by group or by class
methods.* In many hospitals and rehabilitation centres men and
women are exercised together in the same groups or classes.

General Exercises.—General exercises are frequently used
in addition to specific exercises.

THE EXERCISE TABLE

The exercises are selected with regard to the aims of treatment
and the phase of recovery reached by the patient. In general, the
same types of exercises are used for men and women; some of the
very strenuous exercises, however, are not suitable for women.

---

* *Group Treatment.* A small number of patients (6–8 at the most), with the
same or similar types of disability, are treated together. The instructor indicates
the exercise to be performed; the patients then practise it individually.

Class Treatment. A number of patients (14–16 at the most), with the same
or similar types of disability, exercise in unison under the guidance of the
instructor.

One method of compiling and using a table of specific exercises is given here.

COMPILING THE EXERCISE TABLE

The aims of treatment are divided into two groups: those of primary importance, and those of secondary importance (*see* p. 153). The exercises which are chosen to achieve the aims are also divided into two groups: Primary and Secondary exercises. (*See* List of Exercises, pp. 153–154.)

USING THE EXERCISE TABLES

The primary and secondary exercises are used at each exercise period. The secondary exercises are spaced between the primary exercises, e.g., two or three primary exercises are followed by one or two secondary exercises. In this way there is no danger of the affected part being subjected to too concentrated a period of activity. When the table consists of one group of exercises only this suggestion cannot be followed.

Avoiding Fatigue.—Exercises which activate the same muscle groups should not be given consecutively, because this may produce fatigue. Exercises which use the same muscles in association with other muscles, to produce different movements, may follow each other with little danger of over-fatigue. For example, in strengthening the trunk muscles two exercises which use the abdominal muscles as flexors of the spine should not be given consecutively, but a series of exercises in which the abdominal muscles are used as flexors, rotators, and lateral flexors of the spine is permissible. Short rest periods are given whenever they are thought to be necessary.

'LITTLE AND OFTEN' SELF-PRACTICE

To obtain the maximum benefit from specific exercise therapy, the patient should practise two or three of the more important exercises from the exercise table on a 'little and often' basis during the day. Unfortunately, this aspect of physical treatment is often overlooked.

The exercises selected for self-practice must be simple, and— if the patient is confined to bed—capable of being performed with the minimum disturbance of the bedclothes. For example, *Quadriceps contractions* and *single straight Leg raising in small range* are the 'key' exercises prescribed for a patient resting in bed after meniscectomy.

LISTS OF SPECIFIC EXERCISES

To aid the instructor in planning exercise tables for certain clinical conditions some lists of progressive exercises are given in the following chapters. Introductory notes in each chapter describe the conditions for which the exercises are suitable, and give details of the surgical procedures used.

CHAPTER XVI

GASTRECTOMY*

PARTIAL gastrectomy may be performed in the treatment of peptic ulcer (gastric or duodenal ulcer), and carcinoma of the stomach. Total gastrectomy may be performed for: (1) Carcinoma of the stomach; (2) High gastric ulcer; and (3) Ulcer of the lower end of the œsophagus.

TYPES OF INCISION.—A right upper paramedian incision is commonly used (*Fig.* 176). Sometimes a left upper paramedian incision is used, e.g., in certain cases of gastric ulcer and in carcinoma when wide removal of the stomach is necessary.

The incision is vertical in direction, and is situated ½–1 in. from the midline; it extends approximately from the costal margin to a point one side of the umbilicus (*Fig.* 176).

Stages of Incision.—

1. Incision of skin and subcutaneous tissues, down to the anterior sheath of the rectus muscle.

2. Incision of the anterior sheath of the rectus muscle in the line of the skin incision.

3. Retraction of the rectus muscle laterally, so that no large nerves or vessels are damaged.

4. Incision of the posterior rectus sheath and peritoneum in the line of the skin incision.

EXERCISE AND THE SUTURE LINE.—The aponeuroses of the oblique and transverse abdominal muscles form the anterior and posterior sheaths of the rectus muscle. Active trunk rotation movements will therefore tend to pull more strongly on the suture

---

* *a.* A gastro-enterostomy (to short-circuit the pyloric part of the stomach and the duodenum) is performed by some surgeons for inoperable cases of carcinoma of the pylorus and for pyloric stenosis. A right upper paramedian incision is used; the after-treatment is the same as described for gastrectomy.

b. Vagotomy, together with gastro-enterostomy, is sometimes performed for cases of duodenal ulcer with pyloric stenosis and hyperacidity. A left upper paramedian incision is used; the after-treatment is as described for gastrectomy.

6

line than any other form of trunk exercise. When trunk rotation movements are performed they should be of the slow controlled type, and quick, jerky movements must be avoided.

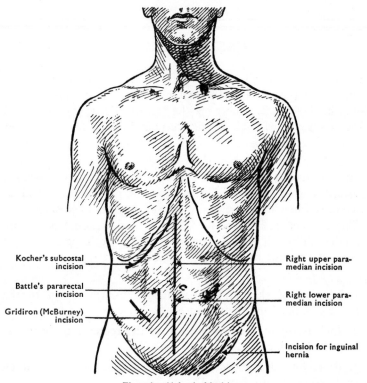

Kocher's subcostal incision

Battle's pararectal incision

Gridiron (McBurney) incision

Right upper para-median incision

Right lower para-median incision

Incision for inguinal hernia

Fig. 176.—Abdominal incisions.

Although it is quite possible (and safe) for the average patient to perform simple abdominal exercises of all types on the 1st and 2nd post-operative days, it has been found more convenient in practice to leave these exercises until the 3rd day. Breathing exercises and movements for the lower limbs are essential during the first two post-operative days, and usually there is little time for abdominal exercises.

EXERCISE THERAPY

The lists of progressive exercises given here are intended to be a guide to the after-treatment of partial or total gastrectomy.

First Two Post-operative Days

Usually intravenous therapy is used on the first day, and one of the patient's arms or legs is immobilized for this purpose. A Ryle's tube is in position for intermittent aspiration of the stomach remnant.

Alteration of Posture.—The patient is encouraged to lie flat on his back and on the left and right side (*Fig.* 177); he remains in each position for about one to two hours at a time. This routine alteration of posture assists in the drainage of the lungs, and is of great importance in the prevention of pulmonary complications, such as atelectasis (*see* p. 159); it also helps to 'break' any flatulence which may be present.

Postural Drainage.—Should a collapse of a particular area of the lung develop in spite of all precautions, the patient's posture must be modified to secure adequate drainage of the affected part,

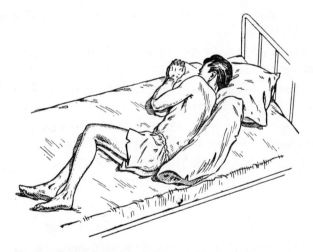

Fig. 177.—Alteration of posture after abdominal surgery. The patient lies on his back and on the left and right side for about 1–2 hours at a time.

e.g., if the lateral area of the left lower lobe is affected the patient is placed in the right crook side lying position (*Fig.* 177), and the foot of the bed is raised 12–24 in. Routine alteration of posture, as indicated above, must still be continued, but the patient spends more time in the specific drainage position.

REMEDIAL AIMS.—

Primary.—

1. To prevent post-operative respiratory complications. (*See* p. 159.)

2. To accelerate the circulation through the veins of the lower limbs and pelvis. (*See* p. 160.)

EXERCISE PERIOD.—Fifteen to twenty minutes, two or three times daily.

Primary Exercises

BREATHING EXERCISES.—

1. Crook lying (hand on upper abdomen); Diaphragmatic breathing.* (*See Figs.* 107 and 110, pp. 77 and 80.)

2. Crook lying (hands on sides of lower chest); lower lateral Costal breathing. (*See Figs.* 106 and 110, pp. 76 and 80.)

3. Crook lying (fists on chest below clavicles); Apical breathing. (*See Fig.* 110, p. 80.)

4. Crook side lying (hand on upper abdomen); Diaphragmatic breathing.*

5. Crook side lying (hand on side of lower chest); lower lateral Costal breathing (unilateral).

6. Crook side lying (instructor's hand on posterior aspect of lower chest); posterior Basal breathing (unilateral).

7. Lying and crook side lying (wound area supported by hand); coughing and expectoration of sputum.

LEG EXERCISES.—

8. Lying; alternate Ankle bending and stretching.

9. Lying; alternate Foot turning inward and outward.

10. Lying; Toe bending and stretching: both feet.

11. Lying; single slight Knee raising and lowering, followed by Leg downpressing.

12. Lying; single or double Quadriceps contractions.

---

* Diaphragmatic breathing is extremely shallow on the first post-operative day (*see* p. 159), and may be almost impossible to obtain.

Third and Fourth Post-operative Days

The patient rests in bed, and—provided there are no respiratory complications—is allowed to sit up. 'Getting up' depends on the patient's condition and age, and the individual opinion of the surgeon. In general, sitting over the edge of the bed, and sitting out in a chair for a few minutes, are allowed on the third day. The time of sitting out is extended on the fourth day, and a small amount of walking is allowed.

REMEDIAL AIMS.—

Primary.—

1. To prevent post-operative respiratory complications. (*See* p. 159.)

2. To accelerate the circulation through the veins of the lower limbs and pelvis. (*See* p. 160.)

3. To maintain the abdominal muscles, particularly the oblique and transverse groups.

Secondary.—

1. To maintain the other trunk muscles.

2. To maintain the muscles which support the medial longitudinal arches of the feet.

EXERCISE PERIOD.—Twenty minutes, twice daily.

Primary Exercises

BREATHING EXERCISES.—

1. Crook lying (hand on upper abdomen); Diaphragmatic breathing. (*See Figs.* 107 and 110, pp. 77 and 80.)

2. Crook side lying (hand on upper abdomen); Diaphragmatic breathing.

3. Crook lying (hands on sides of lower chest); lower lateral Costal breathing. (*See Figs.* 106 and 110, pp. 76 and 80.)

4. Crook lying (fists on chest below clavicles); Apical breathing. (*See Fig.* 110, p. 80.)

5. Crook side lying (instructor's hand on posterior aspect of lower chest); posterior Basal breathing (unilateral).

6. Lying and sitting (wound area supported by hand); coughing and expectoration of sputum.

Leg Exercises.—

7. Lying; single Foot circling.

8. Lying; single Knee raising and lowering, followed by Leg downpressing.

9. High sitting (bed); alternate lower Leg swinging with Ankle bending and stretching. (*See Fig.* 164, p. 136.)

10. High sitting (bed); alternate Ankle bending and stretching.

11. Sitting (chair); alternate Forefoot raising.

12. Sitting (chair); alternate Heel raising.

13. Sitting (chair); single Knee stretching.

Trunk Exercises.—

14. Crook lying (hand on abdomen); Abdominal contractions.

15. Stride lying; Trunk turning with single Arm carrying across the chest. (*See Fig.* 92, p. 68.)

16. Lying; Head bending forward with single high Knee raising. (*See Figs.* 13 and 22, pp. 25 and 33.)

Secondary Exercises

Trunk Exercises.—

1. Lying; slight Chest raising. (*See Fig.* 43, p. 44, which shows full-range Chest raising.)

2. Crook lying; Pelvis raising. (*See Fig.* 112, p. 84.)

Leg Exercises.—

3. Lying; single or double Ankle bending.

4. Lying; single or double Foot turning inward.

Fifth to Tenth Post-operative Day

Usually the clips are removed on the fifth day, and the stitches on the tenth day; these times vary with the patient's condition and the surgeon's opinion. The patient sits out of bed at intervals during the day, and the amount of walking is increased gradually.

Remedial Aims.—As in previous section (p. 153). In addition (Primary): To improve posture and re-institute walking.

Exercise Period.—Twenty to thirty minutes, once or twice daily.

1. PATIENT LYING IN BED
Primary Exercises

BREATHING EXERCISES.—

1. Crook lying (hand on upper abdomen); Diaphragmatic breathing. (*See Figs.* 107 and 110, pp. 77 and 80.)

2. Crook lying (hands on sides of lower chest); lower lateral Costal breathing. (*See Figs.* 106 and 110, pp. 76 and 80.)

LEG EXERCISE.—

3. Half lying; single high Knee raising and lowering, followed by Leg downpressing.

TRUNK EXERCISES.—

4. Stride lying; Trunk turning with Head bending forward and single Arm carrying across the chest. (*See Fig.* 92, p. 68.)

5. Lying; single high Knee raising, Leg stretching forward to 45°, and slow lowering.

6. Lying (hands grasping edges of mattress); upper Trunk bending forward with assistance from arms.

7. Heave grasp lying (head posts of bed); Hip updrawing. (*See Fig.* 84, p. 63.)

Secondary Exercises

TRUNK EXERCISE.—

1. Lying; Chest raising. (*See Fig.* 43, p. 44.)

2. PATIENT SITTING ON CHAIR
Primary Exercises

LEG EXERCISES.—

1. Sitting; alternate Forefoot and Heel raising.

2. Sitting; single high Knee raising, lowering and downpressing of Foot on to floor.

TRUNK EXERCISES.—

3. Stride sitting; Trunk turning with Arm moving loosely sideways in the direction of the turning to grasp the chair back (*Fig.* 178).

4. Stride sitting; Trunk bending sideways.

Secondary Exercises

TRUNK EXERCISE.—

1. Stride sitting (hands on thighs); Trunk bending forward-downward to assume a modified lax stoop position (movement taken as far as possible without producing discomfort in wound area), followed by Trunk stretching (*Fig.* 179).

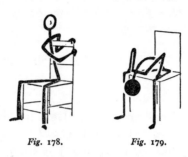

Fig. 178.   Fig. 179.

3. PATIENT STANDING

Primary Exercises

CHECK OF POSTURE AND WALKING.—

1. General correction of posture in standing and walking.
2. Walking practice.

Tenth to Fourteenth Post-operative Day

The patient is often discharged from the ward on the fourteenth day.

REMEDIAL AIMS.—

Primary.—

To redevelop the abdominal muscles, particularly the oblique and transverse groups.

Secondary.—

1. To develop the other trunk muscles.

2. To redevelop the muscles which support the medial longitudinal arches of the feet.

3. To re-educate neuromuscular co-ordination.

EXERCISE PERIOD.—Thirty minutes, twice daily.

Primary Exercises

TRUNK EXERCISES.—

1. Fixed stride lying; upper Trunk bending forward with turning and single Arm carrying across the chest (*Fig.* 180).

2. Crook lying; Pelvis raising and turning.

3. Half lumbar rest stride standing; single Arm swinging forward, and sideways with Trunk turning.

4. Low reach grasp standing (chair back); Hip updrawing. (*See Fig.* 84, p. 63.)

5. Stride standing; Trunk bending sideways.

6. Lying; high Knee raising, followed by over-pressure with the hands, and upper Trunk bending forward. (*See Fig.* 36, p. 38.)

7. Lying; upper Trunk bending forward with single high Knee raising. (*See Figs.* 22 and 30, pp. 33 and 36.)

8. Lying; cycling.

Secondary Exercises

TRUNK EXERCISES.—

1. Lax stoop stride sitting; Trunk stretching 'vertebra by vertebra' in different planes. (*See Fig.* 102, p. 71.)

2. Crook lying; Chest raising. (*See Fig.* 43, p. 44.)

3. Forehead rest prone lying (pillow under abdomen); single slight Leg raising backward.

4. Neck rest stride sitting; Trunk lowering forward.

LEG EXERCISE.—

5. Low reach grasp standing (chair back); inner Border raising.

BALANCE EXERCISES.—

6. Back toward standing (wall bars or wall); single Knee raising.

7. Half yard finger support side toward standing (wall bars or wall); balance walking forward with Knee raising.

From the Fourteenth Post-operative Day

The exercises suggested here are of a moderately strenuous type. They may be used for 1–2 weeks if exercise therapy is prescribed for the patient when he is discharged from the ward.

REMEDIAL AIMS.—*See* previous section, p. 156.

EXERCISE PERIOD.—Thirty minutes, twice daily.

Primary Exercises

TRUNK EXERCISES.—

1. Fixed stride lying; upper Trunk bending forward with turning and single Arm carrying across the chest (*Fig.* 180).

2. Prone kneeling; slow Trunk turning with single Arm raising sideways (*Fig.* 181).

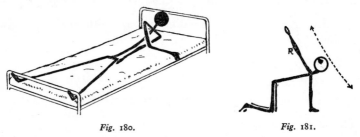

Fig. 180.   Fig. 181.

3. Stride standing; Trunk bending sideways.

4. Fixed crook lying; Trunk bending forward with assistance from arms. (*See Fig.* 35, p. 38.)

5. Fist bend fixed inclined long sitting (wall bar stool); Trunk lowering backward through 45°. (*See Fig.* 23, p. 33.)

Secondary Exercises

TRUNK EXERCISES.—

1. Lax stoop back lean stride standing (heels 12–15 in. in front of wall bar upright); Trunk stretching 'vertebra by vertebra' in different planes. (*See Fig.* 102, p. 71.)

2. Neck rest crook lying; Chest raising. (*See Fig.* 43, p. 44.)

3. Forehead rest prone lying; single Leg raising backward. The exercise may have to be modified, so that the spinal extension does not stretch the abdominal muscles unduly or cause pain.

4. Prone kneeling; Pelvis tilting forward and backward with Head bending backward and forward. (*See Fig.* 69, p. 56.)

5. Fist bend stride sitting; Trunk lowering forward.

FOOT EXERCISE.—

6. Standing; inner Border raising.

BALANCE EXERCISES.—

7. Balance walking forward with opposite Knee and Arm raising.

8. Balance half standing (balance bench rib); balance walking forward and backward.

POST-OPERATIVE RESPIRATORY AND CIRCULATORY COMPLICATIONS

RESPIRATORY COMPLICATIONS

The main causes of post-operative respiratory complications, such as bronchitis, bronchopneumonia, and atelectasis, are: (1) Decreased respiratory movement, particularly limitation of diaphragmatic excursion, and (2) Increased amount of mucous secretions in the respiratory passages, as a result of some anæsthetic agent irritation, and inhibition—for a variable period—of the normal ciliary action.

1. DECREASED RESPIRATORY MOVEMENT.—This means that parts of the lungs are out of action and not expanding fully, especially at the bases. The main factors which produce this state are pain and associated reflex spasm of the diaphragm.

The respiratory excursion of the diaphragm is especially limited after operations on the upper abdomen, and this is most evident on the first post-operative day. Indeed, the fall of vital capacity is reported (Patey, 1930) as being as low as 20–25 per cent of normal on the first post-operative day; after this it gradually improves, and reaches the pre-operative level by the seventh to the twelfth day.

2. INCREASED AMOUNT OF MUCOUS SECRETIONS.—Normally the cough reflex ensures that the patient successfully empties his respiratory passages of secretions. After general anæsthesia, with or without post-operative analgesic drugs, the reflex is very often diminished for as long as twenty-four hours; in addition, the patient is disinclined to cough because of the associated pain in his wound.

Interaction of the above Factors.—Both the decreased respiratory movement and the increased amount of secretions lead to pulmonary congestion and the danger of blockage of a main bronchus, or to multiple patchy collapse by blockage of many small bronchioles. The latter complication is especially likely to proceed to bronchial pneumonia, if inadequately dealt with. Bronchopneumonia, however, may arise independent of collapse, due to infected material (often inhaled from the mouth) gaining foothold on predisposed ground.

CIRCULATORY COMPLICATIONS

"Various factors have been recorded as being responsible for the production of thrombosis and embolism. Three main factors are now recognized as being the probable causes: (*a*) Increased tendency for the blood to clot, (*b*) Injury to the intima of the vein at operation, and (*c*) Slowing of the venous circulation. The last is probably the most important. . . . This slowing starts on the second post-operative day and is present until the patient becomes ambulant. . . . Several competent authorities think that the slowing of the circulation which occurs in the veins of the lower limbs after abdominal surgery is due to interference with the action of the diaphragm. The diaphragm, in addition to fulfilling a respiratory function, also accounts in large measure for the movement of the blood through the veins to the right heart—the pumping action of the diaphragm [by production of intermittent negative pressure in the chest]. As the movements of the diaphragm are much decreased after abdominal surgery, the pumping action is interfered with and consequently slowing of the venous circulation takes place." (Gunn Roberts, 1946.)

REFERENCES

PATEY, G. (1930), *Brit. J. Surg.*, **17**, 487.
GUNN ROBERTS, J. (1946), *J. chart. Soc. Physiother.*, **32**, 58.

Chapter XVII

CHOLECYSTECTOMY

THE gall-bladder is removed in cases of chronic cholecystitis, with or without the presence of gall-stones. Disease of the gall-bladder is more common in women than in men.

TYPES OF INCISION.—The most common incision used to-day is the right upper paramedian incision (*see Fig.* 176, p. 150). In certain cases (obese subjects, for example, where good exposure is required) Kocher's subcostal incision is used (*Fig.* 176, p. 150). This incision was employed more often in the past, before the introduction of muscle relaxing drugs in anæsthesia.

Right Upper Paramedian Incision.—See p. 149.

Kocher's Subcostal Incision (*Fig.* 176, p. 150).—The incision begins just below the xiphoid process and extends downwards and outwards to the tip of the 9th costal cartilage, 1 in. below and parallel with the costal margin. All the abdominal muscles, including the lateral half of the rectus and its sheath, are divided in the same line. The 9th intercostal nerve is severed. Thus this incision produces a flaccid paralysis of certain of the fibres of the abdominal muscles, which predisposes to herniæ.

DRAINAGE.—Drainage of some type is usually employed. In a straightforward cholecystectomy a corrugated rubber drain, 3–4 in. long, may be used. It extends from the gall-bladder bed to the outer surface of the incision, and is retained for about 48 hours. It drains bile secretions and blood into the gauze dressings.

When the common bile-duct is incised and explored (for the presence of an obstructing stone), a drainage-tube (T-tube) is used to drain the common bile-duct. The tube drains into a bottle at the patient's bedside, and is usually retained for about 10–14 days.

EXERCISE AND THE SUTURE LINE.—*See* previous remarks (p. 149) regarding exercise and the paramedian incision. When the patient is heavy and obese additional care is required.

If Kocher's subcostal incision has been used it must be remembered that because the lateral half of the rectus muscle has been divided, in addition to the other abdominal muscles, active flexion and lateral flexion of the spine (as well as rotation) will pull on the suture line.

EXERCISE THERAPY

As suggested for gastrectomy (pp. 151–159). Certain modifications must be noted, as indicated below:—

1. Usually intravenous therapy is not given.

2. 'Getting up'. After cholecystectomy, when a corrugated rubber drain is used for about 48 hours, sitting out is usually allowed on the third or fourth post-operative day, and walking on the fifth day. After cholecystectomy, with exploration of the common bile-duct (T-tube drainage into bottle), the 'getting up' régime is much the same, but may be a little slower. When, because of diminished secretions, the bottle is not required, the T-tube is clipped off and fastened in position. It is usually removed sometime between the 10th and 14th post-operative days.

CHAPTER XVIII

APPENDICECTOMY

APPENDICECTOMY is performed in the treatment of acute, sub-acute, and chronic inflammation of the vermiform appendix. During an acute attack of appendicitis the operation may be carried out before perforation of the appendix occurs, or after perforation has occurred (when a general peritonitis will complicate the original condition). In chronic appendicitis the appendix is removed between attacks ('interval appendicectomy').

TYPES OF INCISION.—The most common incision used in this country is the gridiron (McBurney) or muscle-splitting incision. Other incisions are Battle's pararectal incision, and the right lower paramedian incision. (*See Fig.* 176, p. 150.)

Gridiron Incision (*Fig.* 176, p. 150).—The incision is an oblique one, and runs in a downward and inward direction in the line of the fibres of the external oblique muscle. It is about 2 in. in length, with its centre at the junction of the middle and lateral thirds of a line drawn from the umbilicus to the right anterior superior iliac spine.

STAGES OF INCISIONS.—

1. Incision of skin and subcutaneous tissues, down to the external oblique muscle.

2. Incision of the external oblique in the line of its fibres. Retraction of the external oblique to expose the internal oblique muscle.

3. Separation of the internal oblique and transversalis muscles in the line of their fibres.

4. Incision of the peritoneum.

The abdomen is closed in five stages. The dressings are retained in position by overlapping strips of elastoplast.

Battle's Pararectal Incision (*Fig.* 176, p. 150).—This incision is considered to give "better views, but is somewhat more liable to hernia". (Miles and Learmonth, 1950.) The incision is a vertical one, sub-umbilical in position, and about 2 in. in length.

Right Lower Paramedian Incision (Fig. 176, p. 150).—The incision is used when the diagnosis is uncertain, or when exploration of the lower abdomen (usually in the case of a female) is desired. (*See* Right Upper Paramedian Incision, p. 149.)

EXERCISE AND THE SUTURE LINE.—

Gridiron Incision.—When this incision has been used abdominal exercises will not tend to separate the sutured muscle edges, because the muscles have been split in the direction of their fibres. Nevertheless, reasonable care should be shown in the choice and performance of trunk exercises throughout the post-operative phase of treatment.

Battle's Incision and Right Lower Paramedian Incision.—Both types of incision entail cutting of the anterior and posterior sheaths of the rectus muscle, which are formed by the aponeuroses of the oblique and transverse abdominal muscles. Active trunk rotation movements will therefore tend to pull more strongly on the suture line than in any other form of trunk exercise. The suggestions made on p. 149 regarding the choice and performance of trunk exercises in the after-treatment of gastrectomy should be followed.

EXERCISE THERAPY

The lists of progressive exercises given here are intended to be a guide to the after-treatment of (1) interval appendicectomy, and (2) appendicectomy performed for acute appendicitis before perforation has occurred. It is assumed that a gridiron incision is used.

When the pararectal or the paramedian incision is used exercise therapy is based on that suggested for gastrectomy (pp. 151–159); progress, however, should be more rapid.

First Post-operative Day

The surgeon usually allows the patient to sit out in a chair for 10–20 minutes during the late afternoon, and to walk a few yards.

While in bed the patient is encouraged to lie flat on his back and on the left and right side (*Fig.* 177, p. 151); he remains in each position for about an hour to two hours at a time. This routine alteration of posture assists in the ventilation of the lungs, and helps to 'break' any flatulence which may be present.

REMEDIAL AIMS.—

Primary.—

1. To prevent post-operative respiratory complications.* (*See* p. 159.)

2. To accelerate the circulation through the veins of the lower limbs and pelvis. (*See* p. 160.)

3. To maintain the abdominal muscles, particularly the oblique and transverse groups.

Secondary.—To maintain the other trunk muscles.

EXERCISE PERIOD.—Fifteen to twenty minutes, once daily.

Primary Exercises

BREATHING EXERCISES.—

1. Crook lying (hand on upper abdomen); Diaphragmatic breathing. (*See Figs.* 107 and 110, pp. 77 and 80.)

2. Crook lying (hands on sides of lower chest); lower lateral Costal breathing. (*See Figs.* 106 and 110, pp. 76 and 80.)

3. Crook lying (fists on chest below clavicles); Apical breathing. (*See Fig.* 110, p. 80.)

4. Lying and crook side lying (wound area supported by hand); coughing and expectoration of sputum.

LEG EXERCISES.—

5. Lying; alternate Ankle bending and stretching.

6. Lying; alternate Foot turning inward and outward.

7. Lying; Toe bending and stretching: both feet.

8. Lying; single slight Knee raising and lowering, followed by Leg downpressing.

9. High sitting (bed); alternate lower Leg swinging with Ankle bending and stretching. (*See Fig.* 164, p. 136.)

TRUNK EXERCISES.—

10. Stride lying; Trunk turning with single Arm carrying across the chest. (*See Fig.* 92, p. 68.)

11. Heave grasp lying (head posts of bed); Hip updrawing. (*See Fig.* 84, p. 63.)

---

* This aim is not so important as in the treatment of upper abdominal operations (e.g., gastrectomy), because the respiratory excursion of the diaphragm is far less limited. (*See* Decreased Respiratory Movement, p. 159.)

Secondary Exercises

TRUNK EXERCISES.—

1. Lying; slight Chest raising. (*See Fig.* 43, p. 44, which shows full-range Chest raising.)

2. Crook lying; Pelvis raising. (*See Fig.* 112, p. 84.)

Second to Fifth Post-operative Day

The surgeon usually allows the patient to sit out in a chair, and to walk about in the ward. The amount of sitting and walking is increased gradually. The clips are often removed on the fifth day.

REMEDIAL AIMS.—
Primary.—

1. To prevent post-operative respiratory complications.* (*See* p. 159.)

2. To accelerate the circulation through the veins of the lower limbs and pelvis.* (*See* p. 160.)

3. To maintain the abdominal muscles, particularly the oblique and transverse groups.

4. To maintain the normal posture and reinstitute walking.

Secondary.—To maintain the other trunk muscles.

EXERCISE PERIOD.—Twenty to thirty minutes, twice daily.

Exercises

As after operations for inguinal hernia (*see* p. 174).

Sixth to Tenth Post-operative Day

The stitches, if used, are often removed on the seventh day. The patient may be discharged from the ward on the tenth day.

REMEDIAL AIMS.—
Primary.—To redevelop the abdominal muscles, particularly the oblique and transverse groups.

---

* These two aims are achieved by the patient sitting out of bed and walking about in the ward. Breathing exercises and movements to accelerate the venous circulation through the lower limbs and pelvis are therefore not necessary in the average case after the first post-operative day. In this connexion it must be borne in mind that the bulk of the appendicectomy cases falls into the younger age group, in which post-operative pulmonary and circulatory complications are less to be feared.

Secondary.—

1. To redevelop the other trunk muscles.
2. To re-educate neuromuscular co-ordination.

EXERCISE PERIOD.—Thirty minutes, twice daily.

Exercises

As after operations for inguinal hernia (pp. 175–176).

From Tenth Post-operative Day

The exercises suggested here are of a moderately strenuous type. They may be used for 1–2 weeks if exercise therapy is prescribed for the patient when he is discharged from the ward.

REMEDIAL AIMS.—As in previous section. In addition (Secondary): To promote generalized activity.

EXERCISE PERIOD.—Thirty minutes, once daily.

Exercises

As after operations for inguinal hernia (*see* p. 177).

REFERENCE

MILES, A., and LEARMONTH, J. (1950), *Operative Surgery*, 3rd ed., pp. 441–442. London: Oxford University Press.

CHAPTER XIX

OPERATIONS FOR INGUINAL HERNIA

DEFENCE MECHANISM OF INGUINAL CANAL

THE inguinal canal constitutes a weak area in the abdominal wall. During a temporary increase in intra-abdominal pressure, such as occurs, for example, in coughing and defæcation, there is a tendency for the abdominal viscera to be forced into the canal. The canal possesses an efficient defence mechanism against this occurrence:—

1. *Sphincter-like Action of Internal Oblique Muscle.*—When the internal oblique "contracts—as it does in those activities which tend to force the viscera into the canal—the arched lower fibres which form the roof of the canal contract, become straight, and compress the spermatic cord against the abdominal surface of the inguinal ligament. In addition, the cremastic fibres which are derived from the internal oblique contract with it, and draw the spermatic cord up into the canal to act as a kind of plug". (Beesly and Johnson, 1939 a.)

2. *Valvular Mechanism.*—"The canal is oblique, and, therefore, to some extent valvular, and when the intra-abdominal contents are forced against the lower part of the abdominal wall they tend to push the posterior wall of the canal forward into apposition with the anterior wall. Opposite the area of greatest weakness in the posterior wall—the abdominal (deep) inguinal ring—is placed the strongest part of the anterior wall—the internal oblique fibres and the external oblique aponeurosis." (Beesly and Johnson, 1939 a.)

INGUINAL HERNIA

An inguinal hernia results when the mechanism of the inguinal canal fails, and abdominal viscera escape through the deep inguinal ring, the inguinal canal, and the superficial inguinal ring, to reach sometimes the scrotum or labium majus. The escaped viscera are contained in a sac which is composed of peritoneum and extra-peritoneal tissue.

The hernial sac descends within the coverings of the spermatic cord in the male; its contents may include omentum, bowel, fluid, or loose bodies (from omentum). The most common contents are omentum and small intestine.

Failure of the inguinal mechanism may be "the result of irregularities in the development of the contents of the canal (congenital hernia), or may be due to loss of sphincteric action of the internal oblique from the hypotonus of age or debility (acquired hernia). In the most frequent type, the hernia passes down the inguinal canal. For this reason it is referred to as *oblique inguinal hernia*. Weakness of the abdominal musculature may, however, allow the abdominal contents to be extruded at the other weak area of the inguinal region—opposite the subcutaneous (superficial) inguinal ring. This variety, which does not traverse the full length of the canal, is referred to as *direct inguinal hernia*." (Beesly and Johnson, 1939 b.)

Oblique Inguinal Hernia : Operative Procedures

In general, two main types of operative treatment for oblique inguinal hernia may be recognized. (1) Simple herniotomy, or complete removal of the sac. This is the method of choice in infants, children, and young fit adults, where the hernia is generally congenital and the secondary changes in the inguinal canal still revisable. (2) Excision of the hernial sac, followed by repair of the inguinal canal. This is usually indicated in the older age group (where the abdominal musculature is of poor quality) and in the case of recurrent hernias.

SIMPLE HERNIOTOMY.—An incision is made about a finger's breadth above and parallel to the medial two-thirds of the inguinal ligament, so as to expose the aponeurosis of the external oblique muscle. (*See Fig.* 176, p. 150.) The margin of the superficial inguinal ring is defined, and the cord is isolated. The aponeurosis of the external oblique is divided from the subcutaneous ring along the line of the inguinal canal. The coverings of the cord are then divided and the sac identified. "The sac is transfixed at its neck with a double catgut suture, securely tied off, and the excess cut away. The stretched fascia transversalis of the dilated deep inguinal ring is brought together with two or three catgut or linen sutures." (Miles and Learmonth, 1950 a.)

The wound is closed in three stages. The dressings are retained in position by overlapping strips of elastoplast.

EXCISION OF SAC, WITH REPAIR OF CANAL.—After excision of the hernial sac (*see* p. 169), a variety of methods may be used to repair the inguinal canal. The Bassini operation and the Gallie fascial repair are summarized here.

Bassini Procedure.—The operation aims at strengthening the whole of the potentially weak posterior wall of the inguinal canal by suturing the internal oblique muscle and the conjoint tendon to the inguinal ligament, behind the spermatic cord. This method has been much criticized, and Aird (1957) states that it should be used "only if the conjoint tendon and inguinal ligament lie close together and parallel, so that they may be apposed without tension". If they are brought together under tension, the conjoint tendon may tear, thus losing the desired effect. A further criticism levelled at the Bassini operation is that it is said to interfere with the delicate shutter mechanism of the canal.

Gallie Fascial Repair.—In this operation strips of fascia lata from the thigh are used to close the opening in the posterior wall of the canal, a "darning" technique being employed. ". . . The sutures grasp the edge of the internal oblique and conjoint tendon above and the deep aspect of the inguinal ligament below . . . to form a lattice and ultimately a permanent living graft." (Miles and Learmonth, 1950 b.) Dense fibrous tissue is later laid down over the lattice.

ABDOMINAL EXERCISES FOLLOWING OPERATIONS FOR INGUINAL HERNIA

The scope of abdominal exercises depends on the type of operative procedure which has been performed.

1. AFTER SIMPLE HERNIOTOMY.—Abdominal exercises assist in the functional recovery of the inguinal mechanism (*see* p. 168), and so help to prevent a recurrence of the hernia.

Exercise and the Suture Line.—Because the aponeurosis of the external oblique muscle is divided in the line of its fibres, abdominal exercises will not tend to separate the sutured edges. Reasonable care should be taken, however, in the choice and performance of trunk exercises throughout the post-operative phase of treatment. (*See* lists of exercises, pp. 172–176.)

2. AFTER EXCISION OF HERNIAL SAC, WITH REPAIR BY BASSINI OPERATION.—Abdominal exercises help to restore the strength of the abdominal muscles, and so assist in the recovery of the valvular aspect of the inguinal mechanism (*see* p. 168). It is debatable if the exercises can assist in the functional recovery of the sphincter mechanism of the canal; theoretically this has been obliterated by the repair process. In practice, however, it may be doubted if such function has been completely replaced.

Exercise and the Suture Line.—Much the same attitude towards trunk exercises may be taken as previously suggested. From experience it would appear that the repair procedures do not necessitate a more conservative approach to exercise therapy.

3. AFTER REMOVAL OF HERNIAL SAC, WITH FASCIAL REPAIR.— For scope of abdominal exercises *see* previous remarks.

Exercise and the Repair.—The success of the fascial repair depends on the development of dense scar tissue. Therefore, considerable care must be shown in the choice and technique of performance of all post-operative exercises, particularly in the early and intermediate phases of treatment. 'Getting up' is usually delayed for 2–3 weeks after the operation.

EXERCISE THERAPY

The lists of progressive exercises given here are intended to be a guide to the after-treatment of (*a*) Simple herniotomy, and (*b*) Excision of hernial sac, with repair of inguinal canal by Bassini operation.

First Three Post-operative Days

The patient rests in bed, and 'getting up' is governed by his condition and age, and the individual opinion of the surgeon. Usually the patient is allowed to sit out in a chair for about 10–15 minutes on the third day, and to walk a few yards.

On the first post-operative day the patient is encouraged to lie flat on his back and on the left and right side (*see Fig.* 177, p. 151); he remains in each position for about an hour to two hours at a time. This routine alteration of posture assists in the ventilation of the lungs, and helps to 'break' any flatulence which may be present.

On the second and third post-operative days (provided there are no respiratory complications) the patient is allowed to sit up in bed. He is also encouraged to lie on his back and on either side, as previously suggested.

REMEDIAL AIMS.—

Primary.—

1. To prevent post-operative respiratory complications. (*See* p. 159.)

2. To accelerate the circulation through the veins of the lower limbs and pelvis. (*See* p. 160.)

3. To maintain the abdominal muscles, particularly the oblique and transverse groups.

4. To maintain the mobility of the hip joint of the affected side.

Secondary.—To maintain the other trunk muscles.

EXERCISE PERIOD.—Fifteen to twenty minutes, once daily.

Primary Exercises

BREATHING EXERCISES.—

1. Crook lying (hand on upper abdomen); Diaphragmatic breathing. (*See Figs.* 107 and 110, pp. 77 and 80.)

2. Crook lying (hands on sides of lower chest); lower lateral Costal breathing. (*See Figs.* 106 and 110, pp. 76 and 80.)

3. Crook lying (fists on chest below clavicles); Apical breathing. (*See Fig.* 110, p. 80.)

4. Lying and crook side lying (wound area supported by hand); coughing and expectoration of sputum.

LEG EXERCISES.—

5. Lying; alternate Ankle bending and stretching.

6. Lying; alternate Foot turning inward and outward.

7. Lying; Toe bending and stretching: both feet.

8. Lying; single slight Knee raising and lowering, followed by Leg downpressing.

TRUNK EXERCISES.—

9. Stride lying; Trunk turning with single Arm carrying across the chest. (*See Fig.* 92, p. 68.)

10. Crook lying (hand on abdomen); Abdominal contractions.

11. Lying; Head bending forward with single slight Knee raising.

12. Lying (hands grasping sides of mattress); Hip updrawing. (*See Fig.* 84, p. 63.)

HIP EXERCISES.—

13. Lying; single (affected) Knee raising, gradually increasing range of movement.

14. Lying; single Leg carrying sideways.

Secondary Exercises

TRUNK EXERCISES.—

1. Lying; slight Chest raising. (*See Fig.* 43, p. 44, which shows full-range Chest raising.)

2. Crook lying; Pelvis raising. (*See Fig.* 112, p. 84.)

Fourth to Tenth Post-operative Day

Often the clips are removed on the fifth post-operative day, and the stitches on the tenth day; these times vary with the patient's condition and the surgeon's opinion. The patient rests in bed, and is encouraged to sit out in a chair and to walk about in the ward. The amount of sitting out and walking is increased gradually. The lifting of any heavy object is prohibited.

REMEDIAL AIMS.—

Primary.—

1. To prevent post-operative respiratory complications.* (*See* p. 159.)

2. To accelerate the circulation through the veins of the lower limbs and pelvis.* (*See* p. 160.)

3. To maintain the abdominal muscles, particularly the oblique and transverse groups.

4. To maintain the normal posture and reinstitute walking.

Secondary.—To maintain the other trunk muscles.

EXERCISE PERIOD.—Twenty to thirty minutes, once daily.

---

* These two aims are achieved by the patient sitting out of bed and walking about in the ward. Breathing exercises and movements to accelerate the venous circulation through the lower limbs are therefore not necessary in the average case after the third post-operative day.

1. Patient Lying in Bed

Primary Exercises

TRUNK EXERCISES.—

1. Stride lying; Trunk turning with Head bending forward and single Arm carrying across the chest. (*See Fig.* 92, p. 68.)

2. Crook lying (hands grasping edges of mattress); slow Knee swinging from side to side. (*See Fig.* 91, p. 67.)

3. Crook lying; Pelvis raising and turning.

4. Lying (hands grasping edges of mattress); Hip updrawing. (*See Fig.* 84, p. 63.)

5. Lying; Head bending forward with single Knee raising.

6. Lying (hands grasping edges of mattress); upper Trunk bending forward with assistance from arms.

7. Crook lying; Pelvis tilting forward and backward (range of forward tilt being restricted). (*See Figs.* 42 and 31, pp. 44 and 36.)

Secondary Exercise

TRUNK EXERCISE.—

1. Crook lying; slight Chest raising. (*See Fig.* 43, p. 44, which shows full-range chest raising.)

2. Patient Sitting in Chair

Primary Exercises

TRUNK EXERCISES.—

1. Stride sitting; Trunk turning with Arm moving loosely sideways in the direction of the turning to grasp the chair back. (*See Fig.* 178, p. 156.)

2. Stride sitting; Trunk bending sideways.

Secondary Exercise

TRUNK EXERCISE.—

1. Stride sitting (hands on thighs); Trunk bending forward-downward to assume a modified lax stoop position (movement taken as far as possible without producing discomfort in wound area), followed by Trunk stretching 'vertebra by vertebra'. (*See Fig.* 179, p. 156.)

3. PATIENT STANDING

Primary Exercises

CHECK OF POSTURE AND WALKING.—

1. General correction of posture in standing and walking.

2. Walking practice.

Tenth to Fourteenth Post-operative Day

The patient is often discharged from the ward on the twelfth or fourteenth day.

REMEDIAL AIMS.—

Primary.—

1. To redevelop the abdominal muscles, particularly the oblique and transverse groups.

2. To educate the patient in the correct technique of lifting and carrying heavy objects.

Secondary.—

1. To redevelop the other trunk muscles.

2. To re-educate neuromuscular co-ordination.

EXERCISE PERIOD.—Thirty minutes, twice daily.

Primary Exercises

TRUNK EXERCISES.—

1. Fixed stride lying; upper Trunk bending forward with turning and single Arm carrying across the chest. (*See Fig.* 180, p. 158.)

2. Prone kneeling; slow Trunk turning with single Arm raising sideways. (*See Fig.* 181, p. 158.)

3. Half lumbar rest stride standing; single Arm swinging forward, and sideways with Trunk turning.

4. Low reach grasp standing (chair back); Hip updrawing. (*See Fig.* 84, p. 63.)

5. Lying; Trunk bending sideways with single Leg carrying sideways to the same side.

6. Stride standing; Trunk bending sideways.

7. Lying; high Knee raising, followed by over-pressure with the hands, and upper Trunk bending forward. (*See Fig.* 36, p. 38.)

8. Lying; upper Trunk bending forward with single high Knee raising. (*See Figs.* 22 and 30, pp. 33 and 36.)

EDUCATION IN LIFTING.—

9. Practice in correct technique of lifting and carrying heavy objects (*Fig.* 182).

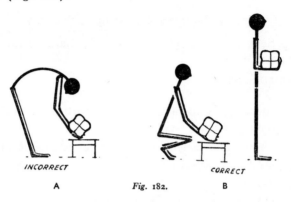

INCORRECT

A   *Fig.* 182.   B

Secondary Exercises

TRUNK EXERCISES.—

1. Lax stoop back lean stride standing (heels 12–15 in. in front of wall or wall bar upright); Trunk stretching 'vertebra by vertebra' in different planes. (*See Fig.* 102, p. 71.)

2. Crook lying; Chest raising. (*See Fig.* 43, p. 44.)

BALANCE EXERCISES.—

3. Balance walking forward and backward with Knee raising.

4. Balance walking forward with opposite Knee and Arm raising.

From Twelfth or Fourteenth Post-operative Day

The exercises suggested here are of a moderately strenuous type. They may be used for 1–2 weeks if exercise therapy is prescribed for the patient when he is discharged from the ward.

REMEDIAL AIMS.—As in previous section, p. 175. In addition (Secondary): To promote generalized activity.

EXERCISE PERIOD.—Thirty minutes, once daily.

Primary Exercises

TRUNK EXERCISES.—

1. Fixed slight crook lying; Trunk bending forward with turning and single Arm carrying across the chest.

2. Turn prone kneeling (one arm bent loosely across chest); slow Trunk turning with single Arm raising sideways. (*See Fig. 95, p. 69.*)

3. Neck rest stride standing; Trunk bending sideways.

4. Wing fixed crook lying; Trunk bending forward. (*See Fig. 35, p. 38.*)

5. Inclined prone falling (hands on beam); Arm bending. (*See Fig. 25, p. 34.*)

Secondary Exercises

TRUNK EXERCISES.—

1. Neck rest crook lying; Chest raising. (*See Fig. 43, p. 44.*)

2. Forehead rest prone lying; single Leg raising backward (limited range of spinal extension).

3. Neck rest lax stoop kneel sitting; Trunk stretching 'vertebra by vertebra'.

4. Over grasp fall hanging (beam below shoulder level); Arm bending. (*See Fig. 39, p. 42.*)

BALANCE EXERCISES.—

5. Balance half standing (balance bench rib); balance walking forward and backward.

6. Balance across standing (balance bench rib); balance walking sideways with heels kept low to let the feet grip the rib.

SKIPPING EXERCISES.—

7. Skipping: skip jump with rebounds.

8. Skipping: hopping from foot to foot (basic skipping step), moving forward and backward: 10 counts in each direction.

REFERENCES

AIRD, I. (1957), *A Companion in Surgical Studies*, 2nd ed., p. 646. Edinburgh: E. & S. Livingstone.

BEESLY, L., and JOHNSON, T. B. (1939 a), *Manual of Surgical Anatomy*, 5th ed., p. 339. London : Oxford University Press.

— — — — (1939 b), *Ibid.*, p. 340.

MILES, A., and LEARMONTH, J. (1950 a), *Operative Surgery*, 3rd ed., p. 468. London: Oxford University Press.

— — — — (1950 b), *Ibid.*, p. 470.

CHAPTER XX

FEMORAL AND UMBILICAL HERNIÆ

FEMORAL HERNIA

A FEMORAL hernia consists of a downward extension of peritoneum through the femoral canal. Usually the hernia is not very large; as a rule the sac contains omentum.

Femoral hernia is commoner in women than in men. This is said to be because (1) the inguinal ligament makes a wider angle with the pubis in the female, and (2) pregnancies increase intra-abdominal pressure.

Men who suffer from the condition usually follow 'stooping' occupations—bakers, stokers, and gardeners.

SURGICAL TREATMENT.—An operation is performed unless there is some definite contra-indication. The sac is ligated and the femoral canal closed. Two main types of procedure are employed, the high operation and the low operation.

High Operation.—An incision is made, similar to that described for simple inguinal herniotomy (p. 169), above and parallel to the medial two-thirds of the inguinal ligament. The external oblique aponeurosis is divided and the posterior wall of the inguinal canal exposed; the protuberance of peritoneum which forms the hernia can then be drawn out of the femoral canal from above.

Low Operation.—A vertical incision, 2–3 in. in length, is made over the hernial protuberance. The sac is exposed, and is dealt with from below.

In both operations the hernial sac is cleaned of its coverings, opened, explored, and the contents (if any) returned to the general peritoneal cavity. The pectineal fascia is sutured to the under-surface of the inguinal ligament. This closes the femoral canal.

Closure of Wound.—The wound is closed in stages. The dressings are retained in position by overlapping strips of elastoplast.

Post-operative Exercise Therapy.—As after operations for inguinal hernia (pp. 171–177). Exercises for the hip of the affected side are important during the first few post-operative days.

UMBILICAL HERNIA

An umbilical hernia consists of a protrusion of the abdominal contents through the umbilicus. If the protrusion occurs close to the umbilicus the condition is known as a para-umbilical hernia.

Adult umbilical hernia occurs almost exclusively in obese women at the end of the child-bearing period. The hernia is probably the effect of increased intra-abdominal pressure (pregnancies, omental adiposity, bronchitis) on the umbilical cicatrix or the linea alba. The hernia sometimes reaches a huge size. It contains usually omentum and sometimes transverse colon and small intestine as well.

Surgical Treatment.—The hernia is treated by operation. Before operation an attempt is often made to reduce the patient's weight by dietetic means.

A transverse elliptical incision is made which outlines the hernial protrusion; it is deepened through the fat until the stretched linea alba is exposed. The sac is defined and opened; protruding bowel is returned to the general peritoneal cavity; omentum may be widely excised to reduce the volume of the abdominal contents; the sac is then ligated at the neck, and excised. The stretched linea alba is sutured transversely with two rows of stitches, so that the flaps overlap; the subcutaneous tissues and the skin are then sutured. The dressings are held in place by overlapping strips of elastoplast.

EXERCISE THERAPY

After Repair of a Small Umbilical Hernia.—As after operations for inguinal hernia (pp. 171–177).

After Repair of a Large Umbilical Hernia.—The patient is usually kept in bed for 10 days to 3 weeks. Great care must be taken in exercising the abdominal muscles, because the tissues are of poor quality and any excessive strain may break down the repair and cause re-herniation. The same types of abdominal exercises are used as described for simple inguinal herniotomy (pp. 171–177), but the time suggested for starting the exercises in sitting and standing must be delayed, as indicated above. In addition, some of the stronger abdominal exercises must be omitted in the early stage of treatment.

An abdominal corset or belt is worn when the patient is allowed out of bed; she must wear it when she first sits out, as well as when standing and walking.

CHAPTER XXI

INTERVERTEBRAL DISK LESIONS OF THE LUMBAR SPINE

WHEN the annulus fibrosus of the intervertebral disk remains intact, but bulges posteriorly, the patient may complain of low back pain; when the annulus fibrosus ruptures, and a prolapse of the nucleus pulposus occurs, then the prolapse may impinge on a lumbar nerve-root and cause sciatica.

Conservative treatment will be sufficient for most disk lesions; surgical treatment will be required for a small percentage of patients in whom the prolapse cannot be warded off the nerve-root.

Conservative treatment consists of (1) rest in bed, with or without spinal traction, for several weeks, (2) intermittent spinal traction, (3) manipulation, and (4) spinal jacket, brace, or belt. Exercise therapy is often used in association with these forms of treatment, as indicated below. Some surgeons, however, do not allow trunk exercises when rest in bed is prescribed.

Surgical treatment consists of the removal of the prolapsed portion of the disk.

EXERCISE THERAPY

When Conservative Treatment is Used

REMEDIAL AIMS.—
Primary.—To strengthen the muscles of the spine, particularly the extensors.

EXERCISE PERIOD.—Thirty minutes, once daily.

Primary Exercises

EXTENSION EXERCISES.—
1. Prone lying; Trunk bending backward with Arm turning outward. (*See Fig.* 48, p. 46.)

2. As above, but with single Leg raising backward. (*See Fig.* 50, p. 46.)

7

3. Fixed prone lying; Trunk bending backward with Arm turning outward. (*See Fig.* 51, p. 47.)

4. Fixed prone lying; Trunk bending backward with turning. (*See Fig.* 101, p. 71, which shows a progression on this exercise.)

5. Lying; Chest raising. (*See Fig.* 43, p. 44.)

ABDOMINAL (STATIC) EXERCISES.—

6. Lying; single Leg raising through 15°.

7. Lying; Abdominal contractions.

ROTATION EXERCISES.—

8. Prone lying; Trunk turning to look over the shoulder.

9. *See* Exercise 4.

N.B.—When rest in bed and exercise therapy are prescribed for the patient, breathing exercises, foot, ankle, and static Quadriceps exercises may be given in addition to the previous exercises.

Posture and Technique of Lifting.—The patient must be taught the importance of not flexing the spine when sitting or standing. He must also be shown how to lift heavy objects from the floor with the spine kept straight. (*See Fig.* 182, p. 176.)

When Surgical Treatment is Used

After the operation the patient rests in bed for about 14 days. The dressings are held in place by bandages, e.g., many-tailed bandage. The sutures are often removed on the tenth day.

First Post-operative Day

REMEDIAL AIMS.—
Primary.—

1. To prevent post-operative respiratory complications. (*See* p. 159.)

2. To accelerate the circulation through the veins of the lower limbs and pelvis. (*See* p. 160.)

EXERCISE PERIOD.—Ten to fifteen minutes, two or three times daily.

Primary Exercises

Breathing, foot, ankle, and static Quadriceps exercises.

Second to Fourth Post-operative Day

REMEDIAL AIMS.—
Primary.—As in the previous section. In addition: To strengthen the muscles of the spine, particularly the extensors.

EXERCISE PERIOD.—Twenty to thirty minutes, once daily.

Primary Exercises

EXTENSION EXERCISES.—
  1. Prone lying (hands under shoulders); Trunk bending backward with assistance from the arms.

  2. Prone lying; single Leg raising backward.

  3. Lying; Chest raising. (*See Fig.* 43, p. 44.)

ABDOMINAL (STATIC) EXERCISES.—
  4. Crook lying; Abdominal contractions.

  5. Lying; single Leg raising to 20°.

BREATHING AND LEG EXERCISES.—
  6. Breathing, foot, ankle and static Quadriceps exercises.

Fifth to Twelfth Post-operative Day

REMEDIAL AIMS.—
Primary.—To strengthen the muscles of the spine, particularly the extensors.

EXERCISE PERIOD.—Thirty minutes, once daily.

Primary Exercises

EXTENSION EXERCISES.—
  1. Prone lying; Trunk bending backward with Arm turning outward (range of movement increased gradually). (*See Fig.* 48, p. 46.)

  2. As above, but with single Leg raising backward. (*See Fig.* 50, p. 46.)

  3. Fixed prone lying; Trunk bending backward with Arm turning outward (range of movement increased gradually). (*See Fig.* 51, p. 47.)

  4. Crook lying; Chest raising.

  5. Crook lying; Pelvis raising. (*See Fig.* 112, p. 84.)

ABDOMINAL (STATIC) EXERCISES.—

  6. Lying; Leg raising through 15°.

  7. Prone lying; Abdominal contractions.

ROTATION EXERCISES.—

  8. Stride lying; Trunk turning with single Arm carrying across the chest. (*See Fig.* 92, p. 68.)

  9. Prone lying; Trunk turning to look over the shoulder.

LATERAL FLEXION EXERCISES.—

  10. Stride lying; Trunk bending sideways.

  11. Heave grasp lying (head posts of bed); Hip updrawing. (*See Fig.* 84, p. 63.)

Twelfth Post-operative Day Onwards

Usually the patient sits in a chair for short periods on the twelfth day, and walking is allowed. The time of sitting and walking is increased gradually. Correct posture is essential.

Gentle flexion movements of the spine are started, e.g., (1) Side lying; high Knee raising, (2) Crook side lying; Pelvis tilting forward and backward, and (3) Stride sitting (hands on thighs); Trunk bending forward-downward to assume lax stoop position.

The patient is discharged from the ward on about the fourteenth post-operative day. Exercise therapy is usually prescribed for a further 2–3 weeks.

Progression.—The exercises in the previous list are progressed in strength and range.

CHAPTER XXII

MENISCECTOMY

INDICATIONS FOR OPERATION.—Meniscectomy is performed after an injury to a meniscus when the diagnosis of splitting and displacement is beyond doubt, e.g., when the meniscus has been displaced on more than one occasion.

TYPES OF INCISION.—

Excision of Medial Meniscus.—Two main types of incision are used: the oblique incision and the transverse incision.

The oblique incision, 1½–2 in. in length, begins close to the inframedial aspect of the patella and extends downwards and slightly backwards to a point about ½ in. below the joint line. The structures involved include skin, subcutaneous tissues, capsule, and synovial membrane of the knee-joint.

The infrapatellar branch of the saphenous nerve may be divided. This causes temporary anæsthesia of the small zone of skin on the anterior aspect of the knee-joint which is supplied by this nerve,* and sometimes persistent tenderness of the scar.

The transverse incision, about 1½ in. in length, is made over the anteromedial aspect of the knee-joint, parallel with the articular surface of the tibia, and about ½ in. above it. This incision does not damage the infrapatellar nerve and provides good exposure. If the incision is placed too low the scar may become adherent to the surface of the tibia.

Excision of Lateral Meniscus.—The technique of approach is similar to that used for excision of the medial meniscus.

ESSENTIALS OF TREATMENT.—Immediately after the operation the knee is immobilized in extension by a firm flannel or domette-and-wool compression bandage; this prevents post-operative hæmarthrosis. A back splint is sometimes used in addition.

---

* "The presence of the patellar plexus implies that sensory overlap is well developed in this region, and it is thus unusual for an area of diminished cutaneous sensation to remain permanently." (Smillie, 1962 a.)

Exercise Therapy: First 10 *Post-operative Days.*—The type of exercise therapy used depends on whether the meniscus operation has been straightforward or complicated.

Straightforward Meniscectomy. — Exercises to maintain the strength of the quadriceps extensor muscle are started on the first post-operative day. Generally the patient can contract the quadriceps muscle statically, although in some cases it may be difficult to overcome the reflex inhibition of the muscle. The aim is to establish unassisted straight leg raising as soon as possible; usually this is achieved on the second or third post-operative day.

Transient pain localized to the site of the operation is to be expected on starting quadriceps exercises. It results from the drag on the incision produced by the contracting muscle.

Meniscectomy with Complications.—Severe pain and reactionary effusion of the knee are associated with certain complications which may arise during or after the operation. Such complications include: (1) Trauma at operation,* and (2) Post-operative hæmarthrosis.†

Patients with a marked reaction of the knee will experience increased pain when they attempt to exercise the quadriceps extensor muscle. The writer is of the opinion that they should not be bullied into exercising the muscle (as is often done), but allowed to rest the limb until the main reaction of the joint has subsided, and a static contraction of the quadriceps can be obtained without difficulty. Straight leg raising will be possible about a day later.

Exercise Therapy when the Sutures are Removed.—The sutures are often removed on the tenth post-operative day, and a crêpe bandage applied to the knee-joint to control œdema. Quadriceps exercises are continued, and intensified.

Opinion varies among surgeons as to when knee flexion is to be allowed. Some consider that knee flexion exercises should not be used until the late stage of convalescence, because in the earlier stages the movements may irritate the joint and produce an

---

* ". . . Cases in which the operation is performed only with difficulty and in which the medial ligament and capsule are subjected to prolonged stretching . . . and the synovial membrane exposed to prolonged pressure . . . frequently suffer from persistent synovitis. . . ." (Smillie, 1962 b.)

† *Post-operative hæmarthrosis.* This may occur as a result of inadequate compression of the knee by the bandage. The condition gives rise to adhesions, residual synovial thickenings, and persistent effusion.

effusion. They stress that knee flexion usually returns by itself without any difficulty. Surgeons who hold this opinion will (in the absence of marked effusion) generally allow the patient to flex the knee within a pain-free range of movement, once or twice daily, about two weeks after the operation.

Other surgeons allow gentle knee flexion exercises (in the absence of marked effusion) between the tenth and the fourteenth post-operative days, provided they are kept within a painless range of movement.

Weight-bearing is usually started some time between the tenth and the fourteenth post-operative days. The patient must be warned not to use the injured limb too much, especially during the first few days. The main factors which control the decision to permit weight-bearing are the degree of effusion present and the stage of development of the quadriceps muscle, and especially of the vastus medialis. Early weight-bearing on a knee-joint which is unprotected by an efficient quadriceps muscle retards rather than accelerates recovery.

Exercise Therapy in the Ambulatory Stage.—When the patient is ambulant the main aims of treatment consist of redeveloping the quadriceps extensor muscle, re-educating walking, and (if flexion exercises are allowed) restoring knee flexion. The reaction of the knee to weight-bearing and exercise must be observed very carefully; any marked increase of effusion indicates that the amount of activity allowed must be decreased and knee flexion omitted until the effusion has subsided.

The length of time required to achieve full recovery after a meniscectomy depends to a considerable extent on the patient's occupation. "Experience has shown that, whereas a clerk can return to his desk in the fourth week, a degree of physical fitness which will withstand the rigours of athletic activities is rarely possible in less than 12 weeks of organized rehabilitation. This applies in equal degree to those engaged in the manual occupations of heavy industry." (Smillie, 1962 c.)

EXERCISE THERAPY

The lists of exercises given here are intended to be a guide to the exercise therapy used after (1) straightforward meniscectomy and (2) meniscectomy with complications.

From First Post-operative Day until Straight Leg Raising can be performed without Assistance

The patient rests in bed, with the knee immobilized by a compression bandage. A pillow is sometimes used to support the limb; it is placed under the lower leg, and does not extend to the knee-joint, because this might cause flexion.

REMEDIAL AIMS.—

Primary.—To maintain the quadriceps extensor muscle.

Secondary.—

1. To maintain the mobility of the toes, ankle, mid-tarsal and sub-talar joints.

2. To maintain the muscles of the lower leg and hip-joint.

EXERCISE PERIOD.—Ten minutes, twice daily.

N.B.—The patient must be instructed to contract the quadriceps extensor muscle for 5 minutes hourly throughout the day.

Primary Exercises

QUADRICEPS EXERCISES.—

1. Half lying; single Quadriceps contractions.

2. Half lying (affected limb supported by instructor: hip flexed to about 60°); single Leg lowering with assistance.

3. Forehead rest prone lying; single Knee bracing, followed by slight Leg raising backward.

4. Half crook side lying; single (affected) Knee bracing, followed by slight Leg raising sideways and carrying forward.

5. Half crook side lying; single (affected) Knee bracing, followed by slight Leg raising sideways and carrying backward.

Secondary Exercises

LOWER LEG EXERCISES.—

1. Half lying; Toe bending and stretching: both feet.

2. Half lying; (*a*) alternate Ankle bending and stretching, (*b*) alternate Foot turning inward and outward.

3. Half lying; (*a*) single Ankle bending, (*b*) single Ankle stretching.

4. Half lying; (*a*) single Foot turning inward, (*b*) single Foot turning outward.

HIP EXERCISES.—

5. Half lying; single Gluteal contractions.

6. *See* Primary Exercises 2–5.

From Second or Third Post-operative Day until the Tenth Day

The patient rests in bed, as described in the previous section. The sutures are often removed on the tenth post-operative day.

REMEDIAL AIMS.—As in the previous section.

EXERCISE PERIOD.—Fifteen to twenty minutes, twice daily.

N.B.—The patient must be instructed to contract the quadriceps extensor muscle for 5 minutes hourly throughout the day.

Primary Exercises

QUADRICEPS EXERCISES.—

1. Half lying; single and double Quadriceps contractions.

2. Half lying; combined (single) Quadriceps and Gluteal contractions.

3. Half lying; single Quadriceps contractions with (*a*) Ankle bending, (*b*) Foot turning inward, (*c*) Foot turning outward.

4. Lying; single Leg raising.*

Secondary Exercises

LEG EXERCISES.—

1. Half lying; (*a*) alternate Ankle bending and stretching, (*b*) alternate Foot turning inward and outward.

---

* When the patient can perform straight leg raising without any difficulty, weight resistance is added, with the surgeon's permission. Usually a weight of 1 lb. is used at first; it is progressed gradually. The exercise must not be allowed to cause pain, or to over-fatigue the quadriceps muscle. Throughout the leg lifting and lowering the knee must be kept firmly braced.

2. Half lying; single or double Foot circling.

3. Half lying; (*a*) single and double Ankle bending, (*b*) single and double Ankle stretching, (*c*) single and double Foot turning inward.

HIP EXERCISES.—

4. Half crook side lying; single (affected) slight Leg raising sideways, and carrying forward and backward to 6 counts. (*See Fig.* 151, p. 126.)

5. Half crook side lying; single (affected) Leg raising sideways.

6. *See* Primary Exercise 4.

Tenth Post-operative Day Onwards for about Two and a Half Weeks: Early Stage of Weight-bearing

Weight-bearing is usually started some time between the tenth and fourteenth post-operative days; the patient then spends most of his time out of bed. A crêpe bandage is worn on the knee to control œdema.

REMEDIAL AIMS.—
Primary.—
1. To redevelop the quadriceps extensor muscle.

2. To restore the mobility of the knee-joint.*

3. To re-educate walking.

Secondary.—
1. To redevelop the muscles of the hip-joint.

2. To re-educate neuromuscular co-ordination.

EXERCISE PERIOD.—Thirty minutes, once or twice daily.

N.B.—Additional time is required for the straight leg raising exercise against weight resistance.

Primary Exercises

QUADRICEPS EXERCISES.—
1. Long sitting; single and double Quadriceps contractions.

---

* Some surgeons do not allow knee flexion exercises until the late stage of convalescence, because they consider that in the earlier stages the movements may irritate the joint and produce an effusion (*see* p. 186). Other surgeons allow gentle knee flexion exercises (in the absence of marked effusion) between the tenth and fourteenth post-operative days.

2. Long sitting; single Quadriceps contractions with (*a*) Ankle bending, (*b*) Foot turning inward, (*c*) Foot turning outward.

3. Half lying or lying (weight-shoe worn on foot, or weights attached to ankle); single (affected) Leg raising against weight resistance.

4. High sitting (plinth: knees flexed to about 30°, with heels supported on stool); single Knee stretching.*

KNEE FLEXION EXERCISES.—

5. Lying; single Knee raising with heel kept in contact with supporting surface.*

6. Forehead rest prone lying; alternate Knee bending and stretching.*

WALKING.—

7. Re-education in walking.

Secondary Exercises

HIP EXERCISES.—

1. Lying; single Leg raising with Foot turning inward.

2. Half crook side lying; single (affected) slight Leg raising sideways and carrying forward and backward to 6 counts. (*See Fig.* 151, p. 126.)

3. Forehead rest prone lying; single Leg raising backward.

4. Lying; single Leg circling.

BALANCE EXERCISES.—

5. Back toward standing (wall bars or wall); single Leg raising to 45°.

6. As above, but with Arm raising sideways.

Fifth and Sixth Weeks of Convalescence

REMEDIAL AIMS.—As in the previous section.

EXERCISE PERIOD.—Thirty minutes, once daily.

N.B.—Additional time is required for the weight or weight-and-pulley resisted exercise.

---

* Not to be used in the presence of marked effusion of the knee, or if the surgeon does not permit knee flexion exercises (p. 186).

Primary Exercises

QUADRICEPS EXERCISES.—

1. Long sitting; single and double Quadriceps contractions.

2. Long sitting; single Quadriceps contractions with Foot turning inward.

3. High sitting (plinth); single Knee stretching with Ankle bending.

4. Low reach grasp standing (wall bars); Heel raising and Knee bending. (*See Fig.* 156, p. 132.)

5. Reach grasp instep support standing (wall bars and stool); single Heel raising and Knee bracing.

6. Lying; single high Knee raising, Leg stretching forward to 45°, and slow lowering.

7. Half lying or lying (weight-shoe worn on foot, or weights attached to ankle); single (affected) Leg raising against weight resistance. *Progress (in the absence of knee effusion) to resisted knee extension: see* Primary Exercise 5, p. 193.

KNEE FLEXION EXERCISES.—

8. Forehead rest prone lying; alternate Knee bending and stretching.*

9. High sitting (bench); single and double Knee bending.*

Secondary Exercises

HIP EXERCISES.—

10. Half crook side lying; single Leg circling to a slow count.

11. Lying; single slight Leg raising, and carrying sideways and across the other leg, and return to starting position.

BALANCE EXERCISES.—

12. Balance half standing (balance bench rib); balance walking forward and backward.

13. Balance across standing (balance bench rib); balance walking sideways with the heels kept low to let the feet grip the rib.

---

* Not to be used in the presence of a marked effusion of the knee, or if the surgeon does not allow knee flexion exercises (*see* p. 186).

Seventh Week of Convalescence

REMEDIAL AIMS.—

Primary.—

1. To redevelop the quadriceps extensor muscle.

2. To restore the mobility of the knee-joint.

Secondary.—

1. To redevelop the extensor muscles of the hip-joint.

2. To develop neuromuscular co-ordination.

EXERCISE PERIOD.—Thirty minutes, once daily.

N.B.—Additional time is required for the resisted knee extension exercise.

Primary Exercises

QUADRICEPS EXERCISES.—

1. Half wing half low yard grasp standing (wall bars); Heel raising and Knee bending.

2. Low reach grasp stride standing (wall bars); Heel raising and single Knee bending. (*See Fig.* 158, p. 132.)

3. Low reach grasp instep support standing (wall bars and stool); single Heel raising and Knee bending.

4. Skipping: (*a*) Skip jumps with rebounds, (*b*) High skip jumps.

5. High sitting (bench); single (affected) Knee stretching against weight or weight-and-pulley resistance.

KNEE FLEXION EXERCISES.—

6. Bend grasp high standing (wall bars); Knee bending and stretching with Hand travelling down and up the bars. (*See Fig.* 168, p. 137.)

7. Lying; cycling.

Secondary Exercises

BALANCE EXERCISES.—

1. Balance half standing (balance bench rib); balance walking forward and backward.

2. Balance walking with Knee and Arm raising of the same side, and opposite Arm raising backward.

3. Toe balance walking along a straight line to 3 counts, followed by Knee full bending and stretching with the knees forward to 6 counts.

HIP EXERCISES.—

4. Primary Exercises 1–4.

Final Stage of Convalescence

REMEDIAL AIMS.—As in the previous section.

EXERCISE PERIOD.—As in the previous section.

Primary Exercises

QUADRICEPS EXERCISES.—

1. Wing standing; Heel raising and Knee bending.

2. Wing stride standing; Heel raising and single Knee bending

3. Wing instep support standing (stool); single Heel raising and Knee bending. (*See Fig.* 150, p. 124.)

4. Skipping: Hopping with rebounds and alternate Knee stretching.

5. Bend standing; hopping with alternate Toe placing forward (and opposite Arm stretching forward), and alternate Toe placing sideways (with opposite Arm stretching sideways).

6. Hopping with rebounds and opposite Knee and Arm raising.

7. Wing standing; hopping with rebounds and alternate Leg swinging sideways.

8. High sitting (bench); single (affected) Knee stretching against weight or weight-and-pulley resistance.

KNEE FLEXION EXERCISE.—

9. Forearm reach grasp kneeling (wall bars); attempting to assume kneel sitting. (*See Fig.* 170, p. 138.)

Secondary Exercises

BALANCE EXERCISES.—

1. Balance half standing (balance bench rib); balance walking forward with Knee and Arm raising of the same side and opposite Arm raising backward.

2. Balance half standing (balance bench rib); Toe balance walking forward to 3 counts, followed by Knee full bending and stretching with knees forward to 6 counts.

HIP EXERCISES.—

3. Primary Exercises 1–7; Secondary Exercise 2.

REFERENCES

SMILLIE, I. S. (1962 a), *Injuries of the Knee Joint*, 3rd ed., p. 161. Edinburgh: E. & S. Livingstone.
— — (1962 b), *Ibid.*, p. 158.
— — (1962 c), *Ibid.*, p. 151.

PART IV

GENERAL EXERCISE THERAPY

CHAPTER XXIII

EXERCISES TO MUSIC, AND CIRCUIT TRAINING

It is an accepted principle that whenever possible general exercises should be used to supplement treatment by specific exercises. Unfortunately, in hospital practice there is rarely time to give properly organized periods of general exercises and this aspect of treatment tends to be neglected.

The difficulty can be overcome by giving the patients a few minutes of 'warming-up' mobility exercises to recorded music before the specific exercise period, and using circuit training for about ten minutes after the specific exercises.

'WARMING-UP' EXERCISES TO MUSIC

The records are played singly, and so only the simplest form of record player is required. Both $33\frac{1}{3}$ and 45 r.p.m. discs are used. Many different types of music may be used (provided it is in strict tempo and is unaccompanied by vocal refrain), from old-time tunes to classical and 'pop' numbers. Some suitable recordings are given here:

$33\frac{1}{3}$ R.P.M.

A Walk in the Black Forest (Herb Alpert and his Tijuana Brass): A. and M. Records.
Spanish Flee (Herb Alpert and his Tijuana Brass): A. and M. Records.
Show me the Way to go Home (Bert Kaempfert and his Orchestra): Polydor.
Bye Bye Blues (Bert Kaempfert and his Orchestra): Polydor.
Midnight in Moscow (Kenny Ball and his Jazzmen): Pye Records.
Sukiyaki (Kenny Ball and his Jazzmen): Pye Records.
Green Leaves of Summer (Kenny Ball and his Jazzmen): Pye Records.

$33\frac{1}{3}$ R.P.M.

Struttin' with Maria (Herb Alpert and his Tijuana Brass): A. and M. Records.

'Warming-up' exercises may be performed in various lying, sitting, and standing positions, according to the stage of recovery of the patients and the conditions being treated. In arranging the exercises it is possible to give particular attention to one region of the body, if this is thought necessary.

Specimen ' Warming-Up ' Schemes

1. *For Spinal Injuries*

The exercises are arranged for use after injuries of the dorso-lumbar spine, during the intermediate phase of recovery. Hyper-extension of the spine is stressed; flexion is restricted to small range movements.

Record: *Bye Bye Blues* (Bert Kaempfert and his Orchestra) Polydor, or *Spanish Flea* (Herb Alpert and his Tijuana Brass) A. and M. Records.

Introductory Music.—

1. Crook lying; alternate Arm swinging forward-upward and downward.

2. Crook lying; Pelvis raising with Arm swinging forward-upward.

3. Stride lying; Trunk turning with single Arm carrying across the chest.

4. Half crook side lying (on left); right Leg raising slightly sideways and swinging forward and backward.

5. Lying; alternate high Knee raising and Leg stretching downward, emphasizing rhythm with heel beat on floor or mattress.

6. As No. 4, but lying on right side.

7. Prone lying; alternate Hand placing behind neck and lumbar spine with slight Trunk bending backward.

8. Prone lying; single Leg raising backward and carrying sideways over other leg.

9. Crook lying; slight Pelvis raising, and swinging from side to side.

10. Lying; Arm swinging to right and left, followed by Arm circling in frontal plane, both arms moving in same time and direction. Sequence repeated until end of record.

2. For Chronic Chest Diseases

The exercises are arranged for use in the treatment of ambulatory patients suffering from such conditions as bronchitis, emphysema, and bronchiectasis.

Record: *Spanish Flee* (Herb Alpert and his Tijuana Brass) A. and M. Records.

Introductory Music.—

1. Sitting; alternate loose Arm swinging forward-upward and backward.

2. Low grasp sitting; alternate Knee stretching and bending, emphasizing rhythm by tapping heel and toe on floor.

3. Low grasp sitting; right Knee raising, Hip abduction, and return to starting position (emphasize placing of foot on floor in both movements). Repeat with left leg.

4. Stride sitting; Trunk bending forward-downward to lax stoop position, and uncurling with Arm turning outward.

5. Stride sitting; Trunk turning to right, and return to starting position with Hand clap on thighs. Repeat to left.

6. Low grasp sitting; raising Pelvis slightly from stool and moving Trunk forward and backward (support of hands and feet only). Forward movement may be accompanied by Heel raising, and backward movement by Forefoot raising.

7. Low grasp inclined long sitting; alternate Ankle bending and stretching (4), followed by alternate Foot turning inward and outward (4), and repeat original exercise.

8. Stride sitting; Trunk bending from side to side with a press in position.

9. Low grasp sitting; alternating between Head bending forward and backward, and turning from side to side.

10. Sitting; Arm swinging to right and left, followed by Arm circling in frontal plane, both arms moving in same time and direction. Sequence repeated until end of record.

USE OF MUSIC IN REHABILITATION CENTRES

In some rehabilitation centres 'warming-up' exercises to recorded music are given for about 20–30 minutes in the morning and afternoon, before the start of the main treatment programme. All the patients take part in the exercise session; they are grouped in sitting or standing, according to their general ability.

A record player which automatically plays a series of records is essential. A wide range of non-vocal recordings is used, e.g., marches, barn dances, and waltzes. (*See* p. 196).

CIRCUIT TRAINING

Circuit training is a comparatively new form of physical education. It aims at the progressive development of endurance and strength, and has a considerable appeal to men and boys. The training enables "large numbers of performers to train at one and the same time by employing a circuit of consecutively numbered exercises round which each performer progresses, doing a prescribed allocation of work at each exercise, and checking his progress against the clock". (Morgan and Adamson, 1957 a.)

In exercise therapy, circuit training may be adapted as an adjunct to treatment by specific exercises, as previously suggested, or used as a separate form of general exercise therapy. The training may be applied as successfully with individual patients as with groups.

COMPILING A CIRCUIT

In compiling a circuit the instructor should ensure that all areas of the body are exercised. Emphasis may be placed on certain movements, e.g., spinal extension when dealing with patients suffering from injuries of the back. Both free and weight-resisted exercises are used; functional activities should also be included in the circuit.

FIXING THE REPETITION DOSE

Various methods of fixing the repetition dose for the circuit are used, and have been fully described by Morgan and Adamson (1957 b). The simplest method is for the instructor to prescribe a set number of circuit laps—for example, three—and fix the repetition dose for each exercise or activity. The patients then endeavour to reduce their time for the three laps. The repetition doses are increased whenever the instructor thinks it advisable. It is important that the repetition dose must be high enough to ensure that on the last lap the patients are working to their maximum capacity.

Specimen Circuits

1. *Circuit for Spinal Injuries*

For use after injuries of the dorsolumbar spine during the intermediate phase of recovery. Emphasis is placed on strengthening the extensors of the spine.

3 *laps.*

Exercises.—   *Repetitions*

1. Fall hanging (beam); Arm bending.   6

2. Squat and Press with Bench. (One end of balance   10
bench is hooked over high wall bar; patient squats at
other end of bench and holds it in his hands at shoulder
level. He raises bench by stretching up whole of body
until he is in stretch toe standing position. He then
returns to starting position, and repeats exercise
continuously.)

3. Prone lying; Trunk bending backward with   6
hands clasped behind back.

4. Lying (hands resting lightly on thighs); upper   6
Trunk bending forward, hands sliding along thighs.

5. High skip jumps with rebounds.   15

6. Barbell squats. (Patient stands erect, with feet   8
slightly apart, and barbell resting on back of neck:
weight-load comparatively low, e.g., 25 lb. With a
quick action he assumes squat position—curtsy
sitting with heels on floor—and returns to starting
position.)

7. Prone falling; Arm bending.   5

2. Circuit for Thigh and Knee Injuries

For use after injuries of the thigh and knee during the intermediate phase of recovery. Emphasis is placed on strengthening the quadriceps extensor muscle.

3 *laps.*

Exercises.—	Repetitions
1. Dodging from side to side under low beam or parallel rails.	6
2. Prone falling; alternating between crouch sitting and prone falling by jumping Feet rhythmically forward and backward.	6
3. Climbing up and down the wall bars: 2–3 bars at a step.	3 times up and down bars
4. Over grasp hanging (beam); Arm bending.	4
5. Stepping on and off balance bench or gymnasium stool.	12
6. Lying (hands resting lightly on thighs); upper Trunk bending forward, hands sliding along thighs.	6
7. Skipping.	30
8. Barbell squats (*see* previous Circuit). Low weight-load, e.g., 15 lb.	6

REFERENCES

MORGAN, R. E., and ADAMSON, G. T. (1957 a), *Circuit Training*, 1st ed., p. 31. London: G. Bell & Sons.
— — — — (1957 b), *Ibid.*, pp. 37–40.

CHAPTER XXIV

RECREATIONAL THERAPY IN THE TREATMENT OF THE MENTALLY HANDICAPPED

RECREATIONAL therapy in the shape of music and movement, games and game-form activities, is a most valuable form of general exercise therapy for mentally handicapped patients in subnormality hospitals. It is capable of wide adaptation and can be used, along with occupational and industrial therapy, as a routine activity for many patients.

THE CONCEPT OF MENTAL HANDICAP

Mental subnormality, also known as mental handicap (and originally as mental deficiency) should "be regarded as a failure to reach full mental growth" (Tregold and Soddy, 1970 a).

In the past subnormality was commonly confused with mental illness. The earliest attempts at distinguishing between the two conditions dates back to the reign of Edward II. A statute of the time refers to 'natural fools' and is concerned with the care of their property.

The Mental Deficiency Act of 1927 classified the mentally subnormal as 'defectives' and recognized three grades: the *idiot*, who is incapable of guarding himself against common physical dangers; the *imbecile*, who is incapable of managing himself or his affairs; and the *feeble-minded*, who is in need of care and supervision for his own protection and for the protection of others.

This classification is still suitable for clinical purposes. The 1959 Mental Health Act, however, abolished the use of the words mental deficiency, idiocy, imbecility, and feeble-mindedness as legal terms.

The 1959 Act also substituted 'mental subnormality' for 'deficiency' and divided it into two grades: severe subnormality and subnormality.

Severe subnormality (I.Q.* 0–50), corresponding to idiocy and imbecility, is defined as a "state of arrested or incomplete development of mind so severe that the patient is incapable of leading an independent life or guarding himself against serious exploitation" (Tregold and Soddy, 1970 b).

Subnormality (I.Q.* 50–70) is defined as a "state of arrested or incomplete development of mind which includes subnormality of intelligence and requires special care or training" (Tregold and Soddy, 1970 b).

The Act recognizes a third condition, *psychopathic disorder*. It is defined as a "persistent disorder of mind (whether or not including subnormality of intelligence) which results in abnormally aggressive or serious irresponsible conduct . . . and requires care or training under medical supervision" (Tregold and Soddy, 1970 b).

Hospital staffs frequently use the terms 'low', 'medium', and 'high' grade when referring to these patients. Psychopaths are included among the high grades.

The World Health Organization uses the term 'mental retardation' in place of subnormality, and has adopted a more elaborate system of classification: profound mental retardation (I.Q.* under 20); severe (I.Q. 20–35); moderate (I.Q. 36–51); mild (I.Q. 52–67); and border-line (I.Q. 68–85).

The term 'mental retardation' is widely used in the United States. It has the disadvantage that its literal meaning implies either some previous period of more rapid development or a delayed accomplishment.

CAUSES

The causes of mental subnormality are widespread. They include: (1) Genetic or hereditary factors, such as metabolic disorders (e.g., phenylketonuria), chromosomal abnormalities (e.g., mongolism or Down's syndrome), and neurological disorders, such as neurofibromatosis (multiple tumours of spinal and cranial nerves). (2) Factors acting in utero, e.g., damage to the foetus due to (*a*) maternal infection, such as rubella (German measles) and other infections, (*b*) drugs taken by the mother, and (*c*) X-irradiation. (3) Factors acting during the birth process, e.g., cerebral anoxia from prolonged labour or hæmorrhage, brain damage from special obstetrical procedures required by malpresentations.

---

* Terman Merrill I.Q.

(4) Post-natal factors. These consist of (*a*) various infections, mainly viral, which the growing child may contact, e.g., encephalitis, (*b*) lead poisoning, and (*c*) severe head injuries resulting from accidents.

Other causes include environmental or social deprivation. The child's capacity to learn and develop may be considerably restricted by a lack of normal emotional or intellectual stimulation. This is particularly so if the child or his parents are of below average intelligence.

Kirman says: "We are still very much in the dark as to the causes of most cases of mental backwardness. This applies even to severe cases, idiocy and imbecility. It is even more true of mild forms of mental retardation. Berg and Kirman in 1959 reviewed 1900 admissions to the Fountain Hospital; the great majority of these were severely retarded children. In only 20 per cent of cases was it possible to suggest a definite cause or to indicate a definite disease" (Kirman, 1968).

NUMBERS

At the present time (1975) there are approximately 61,000 retarded individuals in subnormality hospitals in Britain. A high proportion are epileptic; some are physically disabled (usually as the result of cerebral palsy or spina bifida); a number are blind or deaf. Many suffer from some form of psychotic overlay, which manifests itself in the form of disturbed or bizarre behaviour, and some degree of hyperactivity, e.g., rocking.

Patients admitted to subnormality hospitals in recent years include "a high proportion suffering from severe mental and physical handicap, and they are surviving longer than in the past. At the same time, the number of mildly handicapped who used to assist in the running of the hospitals has dropped. This is probably due partly to the development of community services, particularly training centres, which has made it easier for those with mild handicap to remain with their families, and partly to the success of the hospitals in rehabilitating and discharging more of the less handicapped patients" (*Better Services for the Mentally Handicapped*, 1971 a).

Living in the community and receiving services from the local authorities are some 97,000 mentally handicapped individuals.

Many live at home with their parents or relatives. It is thought that "there may be as many as 90,000 more in the community not at present known to anyone" (C.A.R.E., 1971).

NEED FOR IMPROVED COMMUNITY SERVICES

In the past many retarded children and adults were admitted to subnormality hospitals when their parents or relatives could no longer look after them. Often they did not need hospital treatment at all; they were in need of a home and some degree of guidance. Because of the dearth of local authority hostels and training centres, however, there was literally nowhere else for them to go.

Today, following Government recognition of the urgent need to upgrade the services available to the mentally handicapped, local authorities are being encouraged to develop their facilities. "The services in which the greatest expansion is needed are adult training centres or sheltered workshops, residential homes for children and residential homes for adults" (*Better Services for the Mentally Handicapped*, 1971 b).

THE HANDICAPPED IN HOSPITAL:
BACKGROUND CONSIDERATIONS

The majority of patients in subnormality hospitals are fully ambulant. Many of the adults, however, suffer from faulty posture and poor muscular development: presumably the result of long periods spent in slumped-up positions and a lack of all-round physical exercise. Some are incapable of putting their joints through the extremes of movement; this is especially true of elevation of the arm and extension of the hip. Their gait, too, is often shambling and ungainly.

The doubly handicapped.—Physically disabled children and adults (who suffer for the most part from the effects of cerebral palsy, with spasticity predominating) form a relatively small pocket in most subnormality units. A number are confined to wheelchairs. Some with severe spasticity and gross contractures cannot assume a sitting position without grave discomfort and have to be 'positioned' in various lying positions.

Children from the age of 2–16 spend their day at the special school (now the responsibility of the local education authorities).

In certain circumstances the age limit is raised to 18 or 19. Those who are too physically disabled, or disturbed, to attend are visited on the wards by teachers with a wide experience of play therapy.

The Patients' Day

The adults who are fully ambulant (and some who are physically disabled) spend most of their day in the industrial therapy workshops or the occupational therapy unit. In the workshops they are employed on simple contract work, such as assembling telephone junction boxes, ballpoint pens, and toy kits. If they have insufficient ability to manage this type of work they are kept occupied with play therapy or simple craftwork.

Some hospitals have a range of outdoor activities, such as gardening and greenhouse work, which satisfies patients who need activity of a more strenuous nature. A few possess large-scale 'heavy' workshops with equipment for making up concrete articles, such as fencing, paving slabs, and garden furniture. This is particularly useful for the younger, more able psychopaths.

Work of this sort keeps the patients fully occupied. It gives them a sense of 'belonging' and of being useful members of a working community.

With one or two exceptions, however, it does little to improve their general physical fitness. Too much of any one kind of activity also tends to become monotonous in time. Fortunately the mentally handicapped like repetition too much to become bored easily.

Physical treatment.—Physically disabled patients who are capable of benefiting from exercise therapy are withdrawn from the school and the workshops at intervals, and are treated individually by physiotherapists and remedial gymnasts in special exercise therapy units.

Profoundly and severely retarded.—Profoundly retarded patients (and many of the severely retarded) are not capable of working in the industrial workshops; they cannot achieve the standard of work required and their behaviour often upsets the other workers. Provided there is sufficient staff (and a ratio of 1 to 6 is reasonable) regular sessions of play therapy, using well-designed educational toys, constructional kits, simple jig-saw puzzles, and 'free' painting, are very valuable. A number of the severely retarded are capable of undertaking simple handicrafts, such as knitting, elementary embroidery and papier mâché work. Collage projects are also extremely useful, and a high standard of work can be achieved. Craft and art sessions are organized side by side with play therapy.

Some severely and profoundly retarded patients, whose behaviour makes attendance at the occupational therapy and industrial therapy units impossible, have to remain on the wards. A rumpus room is essential, so that they can indulge in plenty of free physical activity. A separate play therapy centre in the hospital grounds which these patients can attend for short periods each day, accompanied by members of the caring staff from their wards, is also invaluable.

THE CASE FOR RECREATIONAL THERAPY

Regular sessions of music and movement or games are an excellent means of improving physical fitness and providing a complete change of activity. The patients should be withdrawn from the wards and workshops for a set number of recreational therapy periods per week. For each group this may consist of two to three 1-hour periods given on alternate days. The ratio of staff to patients depends on the grade of patient attending the classes, as indicated in the programme section (pp. 220–244).

Whenever possible nursing assistants and workshop instructors should go to the classes, not only to help the recreational therapy staff but to observe how the patients react in a different environment.

For the mildly and borderline handicapped, including those with psychopathic disorders, sessions of games and informal physical education are used in place of music and movement.

RECREATION FOR THE PROFOUNDLY RETARDED: WALKING SESSIONS

For the profoundly retarded and some of the severely retarded (individuals with I.Q.s of below 20 and up to 35) the recreation programme is extremely limited. Music and movement is of little value—useless for the profoundly retarded—however dedicated and skilled the staff.

Organized walking sessions in the fresh air are the answer. During the initial training a good staff ratio is vital: 2 : 1, or 1 : 2, is essential, in order to lay down a habit pattern. Once this is established one member of staff can control a small group of 4 or 5 patients. Obviously there will always be the extremely difficult patient who requires a 1 : 1 ratio.

A walking session should last for about 40 or 50 minutes, although at first the period will be much shorter. Many of the patients will be unaccustomed to sustained physical exercise of this sort; some will be physically handicapped and find walking difficult. Some of the hyperactive, incidentally, will benefit by being allowed to run!

Daily walks.—Daily walking sessions, with the walks varied as much as possible, are ideal, provided there is sufficient staff to cope with the problem. Often it is only possible to organize this form of exercise two or three times a week.

Poor weather, providing it is not raining hard or snowing, should never be an excuse for cancelling 'walking', although some staff need a great deal of persuading over this matter.

On walks the staff should talk to their charges, draw their attention to anything likely to interest them, and endeavour to motivate them as much as possible. Obviously with some patients (if one faces up to hard facts) very little can be accomplished in this direction. But the effort must be made; something may come of it.

Music and Movement for the Severely Retarded

Many severely retarded patients will benefit by taking part in simple music and movement sessions. In general, these will be individuals at the upper end of the 20–35 I.Q. scale.

Whatever form the programme takes it is essential to consider the underlying aims and build the movements and activities around them. Unless this is done the programme will degenerate into a rather useless sort of musical jamboree.

Basic aims. There are 6 basic aims:

1. To provide a period of enjoyment.

2. To cultivate control and discipline in a natural way.

3. To attempt to exploit the intellectual potential.

4. To persuade the patients to work together, instead of in isolation.

5. To improve co-ordination, balance, and body-awareness.

6. To improve the general posture and the mobility of the spine, shoulder, shoulder-girdle, and hip.

Epileptic Fits

Epilepsy, as previously noted, "is a frequent accompaniment of mental subnormality, particularly of the more severe degrees. Major (grand mal) and minor (petit mal) fits may occur in the same patient, and the former may be immediately preceded by periods of unstable behaviour which may occur even if the fit itself is prevented by anticonvulsant drugs" (Heaton-Ward, 1975).

Epileptic attacks may occur during recreational sessions, and it is important that the recreation staff should be aware of the number of epileptics among their patients. They should also know the simple precautions to take when dealing with a fit, and the importance of not allowing the other patients to stop their activities and crowd around.

ORGANIZING A MUSIC AND MOVEMENT PERIOD

Staff.—Music and movement sessions can be conducted successfully by many different types of staff—physiotherapists, remedial gymnasts, nurses, and occupational therapists—provided they have leadership qualities and experience of taking group activities. Whenever possible the leader should be trained in recreational therapy, and it is a great help if he has trained assistants. But excellent work is often carried out by enthusiastic members of the nursing staff who have attended short courses in recreational activities or who have a natural flair for this work.

Whenever possible, the recreational therapy team should be supplemented by nursing assistants and 'trainers' who normally work closely with the patients in the ward or workshop situation (p. 206).

Facilities.—Ideally, the sessions should be carried out in a recreation hall or gymnasium. It is quite possible to run them in a sizeable ward day-room or similar area, although some of the activities may have to be restricted.

Essential equipment consists of a good stereo record player, with audio unit and speakers, and a range of *simple* percussion instruments and games equipment, as outlined on pp. 210–212. A tape-recorder can be used in place of a record player, but it does not allow the leader as much flexibility in arranging his programme. Suitable recordings are given in the section dealing with music and movement programmes (p. 220).

A piano and a pianist experienced in movement offer even more individual scope. Often, however, the problem of finding a first-class pianist who is able to work on a full-time basis proves insuperable.

PERCUSSION INSTRUMENTS

The instruments should be strongly made; they receive rough handling. Those which require special skill, such as the xylophone and glockenspiel, are of little value in these group sessions.

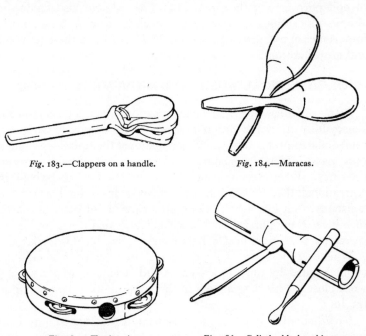

Fig. 183.—Clappers on a handle.   Fig. 184.—Maracas.

Fig. 185.—Tambourine.   Fig. 186.—Cylinder block and beater.

Useful instruments include: clappers or castanets on a handle (*Fig.* 183); maracas (*Fig.* 184); tambourines, 9 in. and 10 in. in diameter (*Fig.* 185); coco-nut shells: one or two pairs; rhythm sticks, 8 in. long, and wooden cylinder blocks with handles (*Fig.* 186); triangles, 6 in. and 8 in., and beaters (*Fig.* 187); motor-horn and rubber bulb; orchestral sleigh bells (*Fig.* 188); cymbals with thongs, 8 in. in diameter (*Fig.* 189); solo cymbals, 10 in. and 12 in. in diameter, and beaters (*Fig.* 190); tambours,

9 in. in diameter (*Fig.* 191); chime bars and beaters (*Fig.* 199, p. 219); Jingling Johnnies (broomsticks and crown stoppers: p. 218).

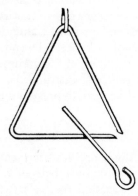

Fig. 187.—Triangle and beater.

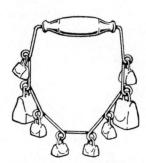

Fig. 188.—Orchestral sleigh bells.

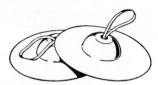

Fig. 189.—Cymbals and thongs.

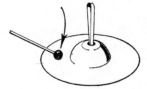

Fig. 190.—Solo cymbal and beater.

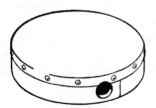

Fig. 191.—Tambour.

Some of the percussion instruments can be made up very cheaply in the workshops. *See Making Musical Apparatus and Instruments* (Blockside, 1969) and *Musical Instruments made to be played* (Roberts, 1969).

INSTRUMENT MANUFACTURERS.—*See* p. 219.

LEADER'S INSTRUMENTS

These consist of a large brass cymbal, about 24 in. in diameter, and a tunable tambour, 14 in. in diameter.

A length of cord is threaded through the hole in the centre of the cymbal, so that it can be hung over the back of a chair. It is used as a 'gong' to start some of the activities and attract the attention of the group. The tunable tambour is used to indicate the end of an activity and sometimes to attract the attention of the group.

Felt-headed beaters are required for both instruments. The beater for the tambour must be round-headed, to prevent damage to the drum skin.

SMALL GAMES EQUIPMENT

Bean-bags of different colours; plastic hoops in various colours, 18 in., 24 in. and 30 in. in diameter; plastic team balls of various colours, $5\frac{1}{2}$ in. in diameter; plain association footballs (white); coloured 'gamester' (perforated plastic) balls for indoor use, $2\frac{1}{2}$ in. in diameter; sorbo rubber sponge balls, $2\frac{1}{2}$ in. in diameter (various colours); plastic pressure pump and inflator adapter; broomsticks: a pair between two patients; skipping ropes (ball bearing); coloured rubber quoits; coloured team braids or bands, 1 in. wide.

OTHER GAMES EQUIPMENT

Set of wooden skittles (Indian clubs are a good substitute); large wooden quoit board and rubber quoits; pair of netball or basketball posts with rings and nets for indoor use; padder bats; goals for five-a-side football.

Equipment manufacturers.—All the games equipment suggested here can be supplied by E. J. Arnold & Son, Ltd., Educational Equipment Suppliers, Butterley Street, Leeds LS10 1AX.

SEATING

It is helpful if two or three wooden forms (balance benches) are provided; they can be used for both the games and musical activities. Square-topped stools (*Fig.* 192) are also useful instead of chairs; they allow a wider range of trunk and arm movements. They can be bought from manufacturers of gymnastic equipment or made up in the workshops. Dimensions: seat top, $15\frac{3}{4}$ in. × $15\frac{3}{4}$ in.; height from floor to seat surface, 17 in.

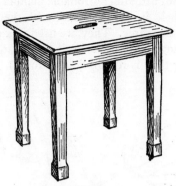

Fig. 192.

PLAYING AND USING PERCUSSION INSTRUMENTS

There is a right and wrong way of using percussion instruments, and it is important that the patients should be taught how to handle them correctly from the beginning. With the severely retarded this is seldom possible; with the moderately retarded, too, it is often difficult. Generally these patients develop their own style of using the instruments, and return to it the moment the instructor has left their side.

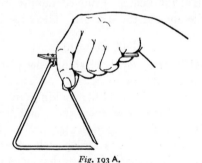

Fig. 193 A.

THE TRIANGLE

This needs a simple wooden holder and a beater. The holder consists of a shaped piece of wood, about 7 in. × $1\frac{1}{2}$ in. × $\frac{1}{4}$ in., with two holes bored near its end (*Fig.* 193 A). A loop of gut or nylon cord is passed through the holes; it must be long enough to prevent the triangle touching the holder, but not so long that the

8

triangle twists about in an uncontrollable manner when it is struck.

The holder is held in the left hand, with the tips of the index finger and thumb kept free. They are used in a pincer movement to 'damp' the triangle after it has been struck, and prevent it from ringing for longer than is required (*Fig.* 193 B).

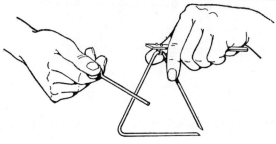

Fig. 193 B.

The beater is held in the right hand with the curled end between the thumb and index finger (*Fig.* 193 B).

A small degree of experiment is needed to find the areas where the triangle should be struck to produce the best ringing sound. This may be on one of the outside arms or on the inside of the base. To produce a trill the beater is moved rapidly between the two arms forming the apex of the triangle. The wrist is kept loose.

THE CYMBALS

They are used in two ways: 'clashing' the plates together, or striking one with a beater or stick.

'Clashing' is achieved by either holding the thongs in the fingers, or slipping them over the hands, and then moving the plates up and down with a perpendicular motion (*Fig.* 194). The 'clash' occurs when the plates strike each other as the hands change position. In holding the thongs the hands must not touch the plates or the sound will be damped.

Deliberate damping is brought about by pressing the plates against the sides of the body after a clash.

Banging the plates together by horizontal movements of the hands does not produce a 'clash', only a dull thudding sound. Sometimes, however, this may be all that a patient who is keen on using cymbals is capable of achieving.

When a cymbal is struck with a beater or a stick usually one cymbal only is used. It is generally held by its thongs in the left hand. A felt-headed beater produces a quieter tone than a stick. Damping is achieved by touching the edge of the 'sounding' plate with the right hand.

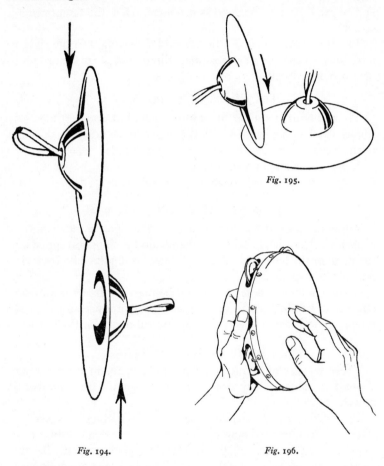

Fig. 195.

Fig. 194.

Fig. 196.

Another method of using a pair of cymbals is to strike the edge of one plate against the outer border of the other (*Fig.* 195).

Cymbals should be of good quality. Thin cheap plates produce a very poor sound, and do not stand up to hard use. The edges tend to dent and split.

THE TAMBOURINE

This is generally held in the left hand, as shown in *Fig.* 196. It is tapped lightly with the tips of the middle three fingers of the right hand. Sometimes, if a very quiet sound is needed, only the middle finger is used. It is important that the right wrist should be loose and relaxed, or a hard sound is produced when the tambourine is struck.

The tambourine can also be played by shaking it in the right or left hand, so that its jingles sound. Single notes can be produced or a prolonged trill.

THE TAMBOUR (*Fig.* 191, p. 211)

The tambour is similar to a tambourine, but does not have any jingles. It is either tapped with the fingers or struck with the palm of the hand. It can also be used with a felt-headed beater.

Note.—Both tambourines and tambours should be stored in a dry place, to prevent damage to the parchment heads.

CASTANETS ON A HANDLE (*Fig.* 183, p. 210)

These are used in two ways: held in the right or left hand and shaken freely, or held in the right hand and the clappers tapped into the palm of the left hand. A crisper effect is obtained by removing one of the clappers.

Castanets on a handle should not be used too freely if a precise effect is to be obtained from the band; they produce an indecisive type of sound which upsets the rhythmical nature of the music.

RHYTHM STICKS OR CLAVES

These consist of round wooden sticks, 1 in. in diameter and about 8 in. long. They can be made up easily from hardwood dowel.

The sticks can be tapped together to produce an excellent staccato effect, or used singly with a hollow wooden cylinder fixed to a handle. (*See Fig.* 186, p. 210.) The cylinder generally has two 'sounds' or notes, one at either end. The handle of the cylinder is held in the left hand and the rhythm stick in the right.

When a pair of rhythm sticks is used, one should be supported loosely between the base of the thumb and the finger-tips of the left hand. It is struck loosely with the other stick. The sound is amplified by the hollow of the partly closed left hand.

ORCHESTRAL SLEIGH BELLS

These are strong brass bells shaped like miniature cow-bells, which are mounted on thick wire and fastened to a handle grip (*Fig.* 188, p. 211). They are among the most useful percussion instruments, being extremely easy to use and giving out a very pleasant ringing sound. Jingle bells, on the other hand, which are mounted on handles or straps, are usually too frail and light to stand up to much hard use.

INDIAN BELLS (*Fig.* 197)

These look like miniature cymbals, each bell being about 2¼ in. in diameter. They are joined together by a short length of cord. In using the bells the cord is held between the thumb and index

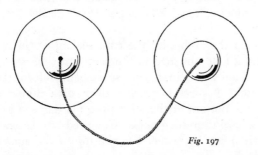

Fig. 197

finger of each hand (close to the bells); either the rim of one bell is used to strike the edge of the other (*see Fig.* 195, p. 215), or the rims are struck together at a right angle (*Fig.* 198).

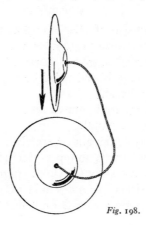

Fig. 198.

The bells give out a clear note, which is attractive. It is only effective, however, in light musical passages, which puts Indian bells among the non-essential instruments of a percussion band.

Coco-nut Shells

Pairs of half coco-nut shells provide a deeper pitch and a greater volume of sound than castanets or cylinder-type blocks. Variations of sound can be achieved by clapping the shells so as to bring them into direct contact, or by adjusting their position so that they overlap each other to a certain extent.

Jingling Johnnie

This consists of a broomstick covered from top to bottom with crown stoppers. The stoppers are nailed loosely to the wood and are free to jingle. The stick is tapped rhythmically up and down on the floor.

To make up the 'Johnnie' the cork sealing of the stoppers is removed and a hole punched in the centre of each stopper. The stoppers are fixed with $\frac{3}{4}$ in. nails, a space being left for the hand to grasp the stick. A piece of thick rubber, or a rubber doorstop, fastened to the bottom of the stick prevents damage to the floor and avoids a hard thumping noise. Coloured 'streamers' (lengths of team braids) can be fastened to the top of the stick to give a colourful finish.

The Jingling Johnnie is described and illustrated in *Musical Instruments made to be played* (Roberts, 1969).

Chime Bars

A chime bar consists of a bar of resonant steel, accurately tuned, which is mounted over a tubular resonator (*Fig.* 199). The resonator is designed to give a sustained sound of a fixed pitch. When struck with a rubber-headed beater the bar gives out a very pleasant bell-like sound.

Some chime bars are mounted on a wooden box frame, which makes them easier to handle.

Chime bars may be bought separately or as a chromatic series of 25 notes, ranging from G to top G, including 10 half notes. The full range is not necessary for simple percussion work. A useful combination consists of 13 notes in key C of the diatonic scale (no sharps or flats) ranging from G up to E.

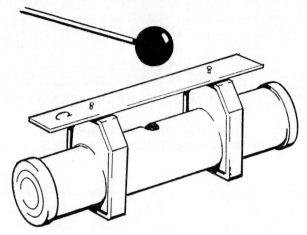

Fig. 199.—Chime bar.

Manufacturers of Percussion Instruments

Two of the main manufacturers of percussion instruments are
E. J. Arnold & Son, Ltd., of Butterley Street, Leeds LS10 1AX,
and Boosey and Hawkes of Edgware, Middlesex. Arnold's supply
direct, Boosey and Hawkes through their main dealers.

REFERENCES

Better Services for the Mentally Handicapped (1971 a), p. 19. London:
H.M.S.O.
— — — — (1971 b), p. 43. London: H.M.S.O.
BLOCKSIDE, K. M. (1969), *Making Musical Apparatus and Instruments.*
London: Nursery School Assoc. of G.B. and N. Ireland.
C.A.R.E. (1971), *The Mental Health Explosion*, p. 3. London: C.A.R.E.
for the Mentally Handicapped.
HEATON-WARD, W. A. (1975), *Mental Subnormality*, 4th ed., p. 72.
Bristol: John Wright.
KIRMAN, B. H. (1968), *Mental Retardation*, 1st ed., p. 7. London:
Pergamon.
ROBERTS, R. (1969), *Musical Instruments made to be played*, 4th ed.
Leicester: Dryad Press.
TREGOLD, R. F., and SODDY, K. (1970 a), *Mental Retardation*, 11th ed.,
p. 1. London: Baillière, Tindall & Cassell.
— — — — (1970 b), *Ibid.*, p. 9.

Chapter XXV

MUSIC AND MOVEMENT PROGRAMMES

1. MUSIC AND MOVEMENT
FOR THE SEVERELY RETARDED

Whenever possible, both men and women should take part in the music and movement sessions. A number of non-ambulant patients in wheelchairs are included.

From a practical point of view it is as well to limit the number of patients capable of taking part to about twenty-five. These form a main 'circle' group. A small number of other patients (often hyperactive or with disturbed behaviour) are allowed to watch: ten is the maximum. They are given chairs some distance from the main circle and form a 'fringe' group. One or two will occasionally attempt to join in the activities; mostly they watch what is going on, sometimes sitting and sometimes wandering about.

The recreational therapist acts as leader and is assisted by five or six instructors. Some will be trained in recreational therapy; others will be nursing assistants from the wards or trainers from the workshops.

The leader operates the stereo unit or tape-recorder (placed at some distance from the circle) and is responsible for setting the pattern of the session. He has to be able to maintain a pleasant rapport with the patients. This is done by an easy conversational style of coaching. Near the stereo unit, hanging by its cord from the back of a chair, is the large cymbal which is used as a 'gong' (p. 212).

Aims of treatment.—See p. 208.

Programme sequence.—The arrangement of the programme and the choice of music is very much an individual matter. A useful method of planning the programme consists of dividing the activities into two main sections. Part 1 starts with a percussion band (for group activity and enjoyment), and includes a simple mime and at least two generalized activities. It finishes with a quiet activity for control and discipline: Sit and listen.

Part 2 opens with two game-form activities. It includes a simple co-ordination exercise (Where's Your Back, Your Neck, Your Head ?), and a generalized activity: Marching in sitting. It finishes with a quietening down activity: Rhythmical clapping.

The programme described here is arranged on these lines and has been used with considerable success for extremely low-grade patients. It is planned to last for an hour. The actual time will depend on the degree of coaching required and the number of items repeated.

SPECIMEN PROGRAMME

(For ambulant patients and those confined to wheelchairs)

 1. Percussion band. *Midnight in Moscow*; *The Green Leaves of Summer* (Kenny Ball and his Jazzmen: Pye MAL 608).
 2. Marching musical chairs. *On the Quarter-deck, etc.* (The World of Military Bands: Decca SPA 18).
 3. Mime: Taking a bird out of a cage.
 4. The stick exercise. *A Walk in the Black Forest* (Herb Alpert and his Tijuana Brass: A. and M. Records AMLS 965).
 5. Mime: Putting the bird back into the cage.
 6. Sit and Listen. Rubinstein's *Melody in F* (Columbia TWO 276), or Dvořák's *Songs My Mother Taught Me* (CBS 30012).
 7. Driving down the motorway (activity with hoops). *Remember When* (Bert Kaempfert and his Orchestra: Polydor BM 56404).
 8. Keep passing (activity with balls, beanbag, and quoit). *Bye Bye Blues* (Bert Kaempfert and his Orchestra: Polydor BM 56504).
 9. Where's your back, your neck, your head ? *So What's New* ? (Herb Alpert and his Tijuana Brass: A. and M. Records AMLS 980).
10. Marching in sitting. *Birdcage Walk, etc.* (The World of Military Bands: Decca SPA 18).
11. Finale: Rhythmical clapping. *Summer Holiday* (with Cliff Richard: Columbia SEG 8250), or *Raindrops keep fallin' on my Head* (with Sacha Distel: Warner Bros. Records WB 7345).

DESCRIPTION OF ACTIVITIES AND GAMES

The patients sit facing inwards in a wide circle on chairs or stools, so that there is plenty of space between them. This enables the instructors to move easily in and out of the circle to give assistance and encouragement.

1. *Percussion band.*—Music: *Midnight in Moscow*; *The Green Leaves of Summer.* This is always a winner as an opening number. Two of the instructors are stationed inside the circle, the rest outside.

The instructors give out the instruments, remembering the individual likes and dislikes of the patients. It is no good trying to fob a patient off with a triangle when he prefers a pair of cymbals.

Meanwhile the leader is spinning his record and announcing to the circle (eager to be off) that they must listen to the music and be quiet. "Listen," he repeats. "And now . . . begin!" giving the gong a substantial thump with his felt-headed beater.

As one the circle tackle their instruments with gusto, often drowning Kenny Ball and his Jazzmen in their efforts to be heard. From time to time the leader raises and lowers the volume of the music, commanding loud and soft percussion (which does not always come off), and a variety of instrument positions: high above the head, at floor level, and in front of the chest.

At the end of the session one or two patients should be asked the names and colours of their instruments. The group is then invited to try a repeat performance, even better than before, with new music.

When this is finished the instructors collect in the instruments (often relinquished with great reluctance) and the group gets ready for the next activity.

2. *Marching musical chairs.*—Music: *On the Quarter-deck.* For this the ambulant patients stand up and turn their chairs round so that they face outwards. They then sit down, with the instructors hovering around the outside of the circle, waiting for the leader's commands. The non-ambulant patients have their chairs turned round for them.

The leader, with one hand on the stereo volume control, says: "When you hear the marching music, start clapping. When you hear the gong"—and he taps his cymbal—"start marching round the chairs. And when the music stops, sit down anywhere you like. Ready . . . ?" And the next second the Coldstream Guards are with us in person, belting out *On the Quarter-deck* as if they were marching down the Mall.

The staff are fully occupied after this, for several of the patients need help in getting up from their chairs and the blind must be guided round the circle. Blind patients usually prefer to walk behind an instructor with their hands resting on his shoulders. In this way they have complete confidence. Chair-bound patients are encouraged to clap rhythmically.

The marching usually lasts for about two minutes. Finding a chair and sitting down is often a longer business; quite a few of the patients persist in wandering around until they find their original chair—only to discover that someone else is sitting in it.

Usually about three or four marching sequences are used. Stress is laid on standing 'tall' and straight and swinging the arms like a soldier, the instructors giving very clear demonstrations.

3. *Mime*: *Taking a bird out of a cage*.—The mime is carried out without music. The leader says: "Now we're going to let our birds out of their cages. We've done this before. Remember? Show me where your cage is," holding up his arms. "Is it a long cage . . . a tall cage . . . or a very small cage?"—measuring with his hands. And when the patients (prompted if necessary by their instructors) get down to the shape of their cages—"Open the door with your left hand—your *left*," as most use their right. "Put in your other hand. Get your bird on a finger. Bring him out and say, 'Good-morning, bird. Nice to see you again.'"

When all this has been accomplished satisfactorily (and it takes time) he adds: "Now let your bird fly up to the ceiling. Give your hand a little shake to set it off. And watch where it goes."

Few of the patients are capable of achieving a complete sequence without prompting. Many, however, remember the words used and repeat them with relish. At the end of the mime some of the patients should be asked by the therapist and instructors to point out where their birds are flying. Other ways of stimulating interest include direct questions, such as "What's your bird's name, James? What colour was your budgie, Maureen?"

4. *The stick exercise*.—Music: *A Walk in the Black Forest*. This is always a great favourite with the patients.

The chairs are moved by the patients and staff until they are in two parallel rows, each chair directly opposite another. The patients sit down and the instructors issue each facing pair with a couple of broomsticks. They hold the ends in their hands so that they are linked together.

The leader tells them to listen to the music and get the rhythm. He then sounds the gong . . . and the patients move their sticks rhythmically backwards and forwards in time. Some find this difficult to do; a few let their sticks fall on the floor and make no attempt to retrieve them. Others work extremely well.

Simple variations consist of 'clapping' the sticks together in time to the music, and lifting one stick vertically and tapping the floor. Often floor tapping becomes pounding. Another variation consists of the instructor striking the tambour and cutting the music—whereupon the patients 'freeze' into statues. A touch on the gong, a re-emergence of the music, and their movement starts again.

At the end of the activity the sticks are collected in by the instructors and tied into a bundle.

5. *Mime*: *Putting the bird back into the cage.*—Keeping their previous positions the patients are asked to look up to the ceiling and spot their birds. They are then told to raise the right (or left) hand with the middle finger extended, and wait for their bird to fly down. With a 'bird' on his finger the leader then shows them how to open the cage door, put the bird back on its perch, and then shut it again.

He says to the group, "Be very careful about shutting the door. There's a cat around." Later, when all has been accomplished, "What sort of cat do you think it is ? A black and white one ? A ginger one ? What sort of noise does it make ? Show me. . .."

6. *Sit and listen.*—Music: Rubinstein's *Melody in F*, or Dvořák's *Songs My Mother Taught Me.* The chairs are moved into a wide circle formation again with the seats facing inwards. The staff and patients then sit down and listen to a piece of light classical music.

The aim is not only to introduce the patients to some good music but to bring about control in a natural manner. After a time the patients will themselves shush anyone who starts to talk or fidgets badly.

Sit and Listen gives the staff a chance, too, of sitting down for a few minutes and getting up steam for the second part of the programme.

In general, the patients prefer orchestral pieces; solo instruments, however superbly played, seldom have the same appeal. One or two patients, however, may be keen on piano recordings.

It is well worth experimenting with different kinds of music. *Melody in F*, the *Waltz* from Act 2 of *Faust*, Dvořák's *Humoresque*, and Chopin's *Nocturne in E flat* are always well received. Pieces such as *Clair de Lune* and Saint-Saëns *The Swan* seem to have a limited appeal.

7. *Driving down the motorway* (*activity with hoops*).—Music: *Remember When?* This is a simple but extremely effective activity with background music. The hoops are held horizontally.

Two or three instructors (depending on the number of patients) stand in the circle, each holding a hoop about 18 in. to 20 in. in diameter: this represents a driving-wheel. They should be stationed well apart and stand directly in front of a patient.

When the music starts each instructor turns his hoop in his hands and encourages the patient in front of him to grasp it and turn it, too, as if driving. Usually one or two complete revolutions are attempted. The instructors move round the circle from patient to patient, so that they all get a chance of manipulating the hoop. Many of the patients who lack dexterity find this difficult, particularly those who handle the hoop with forearms supinated.

At intervals the music is 'cut' and the tambour sounded. This indicates that emergency braking is required: the patients stop turning the hoops, thrust out a foot and stamp down hard on the 'brake'. When the music starts again 'driving' is resumed.

The activity produces considerable movement and enjoyment. At the end (which usually coincides with a braking episode) the patients are asked whether they stopped at a town (useful to suggest one known to them) and what they did there. Did they look round the shops? Did they buy anything?

"What did you get, John?—a glass of beer! You did well to drive home. . . . And you, Anne? You bought a budgie? What colour is it?" And so on.

8. *Keep passing* (*activity with balls, beanbag, and quoit*).—Music: *Bye Bye Blues*. The patients sit in the same circle formation as before, and pass round a number of different-shaped objects: 2 or 3 balls of different colours and sizes, a beanbag, and a quoit. The passing should be continuous and is done in a clockwise or anti-clockwise direction.

Three or more instructors stand in the circle and help with the passing process. This is very necessary; some of the patients fail to understand what they have to do and just sit with the ball or beanbag or quoit in their hands and let it fall on to the floor. Others are reluctant to pass it to the next patient and have to be persuaded to do so. Sometimes two items arrive at one patient and help is needed to sort out his dilemma.

To get off to a good start it is best to begin the passing at different points of the circle, choosing the more able patients as the first recipients. Thus, a ball can be given to patient A, another to patient D, a quoit to patient G, and a beanbag to patient J (*Fig.* 200).

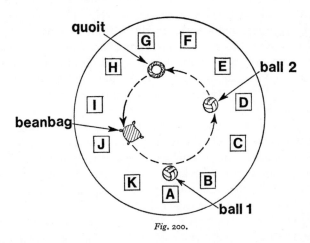

Fig. 200.

The music is kept to a reasonable background level. From time to time it is cut and the leader sounds his tambour. This is the signal for those about to pass to hold their trophies up high above their heads. When the music starts again passing is resumed.

When the tambour halts the activity it is useful for the leader to ask the patients in 'possession' to tell him what they are holding, and give him the colour. It is also useful to ask, "Is it rough or smooth?"

A good finish to Keep Passing is for one of the instructors (who holds a large cardboard box or games equipment hamper) to stand in the middle of the circle. He invites those holding a ball or a beanbag or a quoit to throw it into the box.

He needs to be agile. Some of the patients have little idea of aim of distance, and the box often has to move over to them. A few, however, manage very well and need little help.

9. *Where's your back, your neck, your head?*—Music: *So What's New?* This is a popular short activity, which involves the

staff in plenty of vigorous demonstration. Two of the instructors stand in the centre of the circle and the others outside. One of the instructors leads the sequence of movement and gives the commands.

When the music is played in, and the gong struck, the patients are instructed to clap their hands together in a 'floppy' manner to four counts, the arm movements being made as wide as possible. The arms are then carried backwards and the backs of the hands placed against the lumbar spine: to four counts. Thus: "One, and two, and three, and four. . . . Hands . . . behind . . . the back . . . they go."

Floppy clapping is resumed to four counts, and the arms carried backwards and the palms placed against the back of the neck to four counts. Clapping is then carried out again to four counts, and the palms of the hands placed on top of the head with the elbows kept well back, to four counts.

The sequence of movement is repeated rhythmically in a continuous manner. At first, the clapping and hand-placings are often difficult to synchronize properly. Good chanting style commands are needed from the instructor, as indicated. He and his colleague in the circle must demonstrate clearly what has to be done. The volume of the music follows the commands, being boosted for the clapping and reduced for the hand-placings. The hand-placing sequence suggested here need not, of course, be followed; the instructor varies it as he wishes.

The instructors outside the circle check up on the patients' performances and help those who cannot manage the hand-placings accurately or who get the sequence muddled.

10. *Marching in sitting.*—Music: *Birdcage Walk.* The activity starts with the patients raising and lowering their legs alternately to the marching rhythm. Later they are asked to raise and lower the arms in turn with the legs: thus, left thigh raised with opposite arm, followed by right thigh and left arm.

Two or three instructors stand inside the circle, and are stationed at different points. One is responsible for giving the commands and for demonstrating. The others give assistance to those who find the movements difficult or who cannot get the co-ordination right. Often an instructor finds it helpful to kneel in front of the patient and move his legs up and down manually. The instructors outside the circle can help with the arm movements.

Marching in sitting is always enthusiastically carried out. Indeed, the leader at the stereo unit has to plead for gentle marching. Heavy stamping on the floor can cause the pick-up arm to jump a couple of grooves and scratch the record surface badly.

11. *Finale*: *Rhythmical clapping.*—Music: *Summer Holiday* or *Raindrops keep fallin' on my Head*. This is always a useful finale. The leader, varying the volume control of the stereo unit, calls for loud clapping, soft clapping, clapping above the head, at floor level, in front of the chest and from side to side.

Two or three of the instructors work inside the circle, the others outside.

When the music finishes and the leader announces, "Well, that's where we've got to finish today," he is invariably met with a loud, "Oh, no-oo", from several of the circle members.

2. MUSIC AND MOVEMENT
FOR THE MODERATELY RETARDED

Both men and women take part in the same session. They will all be fully ambulant, with the exception of the occasional physically disabled patient in a wheelchair who looks on and joins in the activities which are within his scope.

The number taking part is best limited to about 26. The recreational therapist acts as leader and is assisted by 3 instructors (p. 220). He operates the stereo unit or tape-recorder, which is placed at one end of the recreation hall. He uses an easy conversational style of coaching, so that the atmosphere of the session is relaxed and informal.

Aims of treatment.—See p. 208.

Programme sequence.—The programme should contain a fairly high proportion of games and free activities with simple equipment, such as hoops and balls. It is important to start off with an activity which is easy and enjoyable and gets everyone moving. The middle section should have a quiet period; for example, Sit and listen or a simple mime. The final item should get the group working without too much strenuous activity.

SPECIMEN PROGRAMME
(*For ambulant patients*)

1. Marching: (*a*) with a long rope; (*b*) 'tall', 'slumpy', loudly, softly, on tip-toe; (*c*) walking in the dark. *Stars and Stripes Forever, Washington Post*, etc. (*Sousa the Great*: Columbia TWO 113).

2. Minor team game: Moving statues.
3. Hoop movements: (*a*) bowling (partners); (*b*) circling: partners linking hands or working independently; (*c*) hoop swinging (partners). *Remember When* (Bert Kaempfert and his Orchestra: Polydor BM 56504).
4. Group game: Centre-circle pass ball.
5. The stick exercise: variations. *A Walk in the Black Forest* (Herb Alpert and his Tijuana Brass: A. and M. Records AMLS 965).
6. Sit and listen. *Waltz* from Act 2, *Faust*, or Chopin's *Nocturne in E flat* (Columbia TWO 315).
7. Ball practice: (*a*) pat bouncing on the spot, and while moving; (*b*) passing between partners; (*c*) tossing up and catching.
8. Mime: Ghosts and watchers. Sibelius's *Valse Triste* (HMV ASD 2272).
9. Activity with a hoop—'Anything you like . . .' Ravel's *Bolero* (RCA VICS 1323).
10. Percussion band. Variations: (*a*) group playing; (*b*) section playing; (*c*) standing and sitting; (*d*) walking round the circle. *Spanish Flea* (Herb Alpert and his Tijuana Brass: A. and M. Records AMLS 965).

DESCRIPTION OF ACTIVITIES AND GAMES

1. *Marching*: (*a*) with a long rope; (*b*) 'tall', 'slumpy', loudly, softly, on tip-toe; (*c*) walking in the dark. Music: *Stars and Stripes Forever, Washington Post*, etc.

a. Marching or walking with a long rope.—The patients are positioned in file, with a gap of at least six feet between each individual. With the left hand they hold on to a long length of sisal rope (which runs the entire length of the group), so that they are all linked together. It is advisable for one instructor to be at the head of the group, and another at the rear, both holding the rope.

The leader tells the patients to listen to the marching music, to get the rhythm. He then sounds the gong, increases the volume of the music, and the group start marching around the hall, keeping the rope under an even tension and swinging the right arm vigorously.

When the gong is struck again the patients swing the rope overhead, while continuing to march, and take it in the right hand. The left arm is then swung vigorously as the marching continues.

Constant coaching is needed from the instructors, who not only have to see that the patients hold themselves upright and swing the free arm properly, but maintain the rope at an even tension and do not allow it to become slack.

Marching with a rope usually lasts for about three or four minutes, with some five or six overhead rope changes.

9

b. Marching or walking: '*tall*', '*slumpy*', *loudly*, *softly*, *on tip-toe.*—Against a background of marching music, at low volume, the leader explains to the group that they are to march or walk freely round the hall. They must be ready to change their style of marching or walking as he directs.

Thus they may start by being instructed to march 'tall'— "Reach with your head to the ceiling. Grow tall . . ."—while swinging their arms vigorously.

After a short period they are told to change to 'slumpy' walking, in which the trunk is allowed to flop forwards and the hips and knees to flex. After this they are instructed to straighten up and march very firmly, making as much noise with the feet as possible.

The next instruction reverses this, and the patients are told to march or walk very very softly, making no noise at all. This leads on naturally to tip-toe walking with long strides.

The instructors follow the commands, demonstrating clearly; they mix with the patients, so that there is no confusion about the change of activity. As before, it is often advisable for one instructor to head the group and another to bring up the rear.

Many other variations are possible. For example, "We're going to march like they do in Russia." "Now we're going to march very slowly and solemnly. Yes, it's a funeral march. You've got to look sad."

c. Walking in the dark.—This needs a soft background of marching music. The leader asks the patients to imagine that they are in the dark, trying to walk across a room. When they have grasped the idea (stretching out their arms and taking hesitant steps) he tells them to imagine that having walked so far in safety, they suddenly collide with a bed or a big chest-of-drawers. "Show me what you would do if your foot hit it. . . ." Some patients put up a good showing, others fail to grasp what is required and have to be helped.

2. *Minor team game*: *Moving statues* (*gong and tambour*).—A very popular activity. The group is divided into two teams, who wear coloured bands. The instructors form part of each team.

Sideways statues.—The teams are formed into two parallel lines, facing the leader, with a distance of about six or eight feet between the lines. The members of each team either grasp hands or link arms, placing them over the shoulders.

When the gong is struck the teams move to the left—indicated by the leader, who not only says "Over to the left . . .", but points out the direction. As they move sideways the leader (who has taken up the tambour and beater) watches closely. The teams also watch him.

When the end member of a team reaches the wall he touches it with his outstretched hand, and the team moves rapidly over to the right to repeat the manœuvre. The moment the tambour is struck—and this must be done as surreptitiously as possible—the two teams 'freeze' into statues.

Anyone who is late in 'freezing' and is caught moving is disqualified. The leader points to him with his beater and indicates that he should sit in the 'out' area. Often only one patient is caught moving, sometimes several. An instructor being pronounced 'out' is a fillip to the patients' morale.

The activity is started again as quickly as possible, the gong being used as the starting symbol. As the teams lose players the action quickens.

The activity is repeated until there is only one member of a team left—the winner. If the game appears to be dragging (a rare occurrence) the leader can be more severe in his judgement.

Forward and backward statues.—This is played in the same way, with the exception that the members of each team are arranged in file, facing the leader, who stands some distance away against an end wall. Each player places his hands on the shoulders of the player in front. Often an instructor heads each team; it is helpful if one brings up the rear, too.

When the gong is struck the teams move forward towards the facing wall. The leading players touch the wall with outstretched hands and the teams move backward as rapidly as possible. When they near the rear wall the end player touches it with a hand, and the team moves forward again.

The tambour is used to halt the action, and the gong to restart it, as before.

3. *Hoop movements*: (*a*) *bowling* (*partners*); (*b*) *circling*: *partners linking hands or working individually*; (*c*) *hoop swinging* (*partners*). Music: *Remember When.*

a. Free bowling practice.—The group is divided up into partners of more or less equal ability. Each pair has a large hoop, 30 in.

in diameter, and practises bowling it forwards and backwards continuously, without letting it fall on its side. The distance between partners is gradually increased. A variation of this consists of each pair getting the hoop in motion and then rapidly changing places.

b. Circling the hoop: partners linking hands.—Each pair is given a hoop about 18–24 in. in diameter. It is circled continuously between them, on extended arms. One slips it on to his right arm and grasps his partner's left hand; they then endeavour to keep the hoop circling in a continuous manner.

Those who manage this successfully try circling the hoop in the opposite direction, stopping it, and restarting again. Another variation consists of the partners moving freely about the hall while they keep the hoop circling. Care has to be taken that there are not too many collisions, which can cause trouble!

c. Hoop swinging (partners).—Each pair is given a large hoop about 30 in. in diameter. They stand well apart, with legs astride, and hold the hoop between them. The hands must be kept at least shoulder-width apart: there is a tendency for the patients to grasp the hoop with the hands close together.

When the gong sounds, and the background music is increased in volume, the partners swing the hoop rhythmically from side to side, then in a sideways–upward direction, and finally in a large circling movement. The leader and the instructors coach: "Swing left and right . . . keep the hoop level. Now sideways–upwards . . . left and right. And now a *big-g* circle . . . starting to the left." All the movements must be performed in a smooth continuous manner.

4. *Group game: Centre-circle pass ball.*—The patients are divided into two groups. Each group sits in circle formation: square-topped stools being used to allow full movement of the body. (*See Fig.* 192, p. 213.) There must be good spacing between the stools.

One player (1) stands in the centre of the circle, with the other players facing him. Player 1 and one of the circle players (2) both hold a ball: usually a football.

At a signal player 2 passes his ball to the next player, who passes it to the next, and so on, the ball moving continuously in an anticlockwise direction round the circle. After a brief pause player

1 in the centre throws his ball to player 2, who throws it back to him. Player 1 then throws the ball to player 3 (who returns it), and so on, round the circle in a continuous anti-clockwise manner, as indicated in *Fig.* 201.

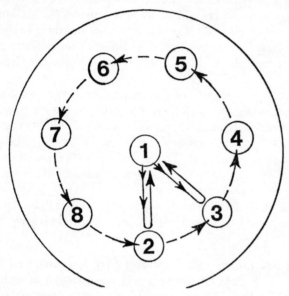

Fig. 201.

When a player receives both balls at the same time, he and player 1 change places. The game is then resumed, the direction of the passing being changed to clockwise.

The two groups work independently of each other, and so it is necessary for each group to have an instructor who coaches the game and gives the signal to stop and start. Usually this is by command, sometimes by whistle.

5. *The stick exercise.*—Music: *A Walk in the Black Forest.* This is an advanced version of the activity described in the previous programme (p. 223), and is extremely popular with both patients and staff.

The patients stand in two parallel rows, partners facing each other, and are given a pair of broomsticks. They hold the ends in their hands, so that they are linked together. It is important that there should be adequate space between the patients.

The leader tells them to listen to the music and get the rhythm. He then sounds the gong, and the patients move their sticks rhythmically forwards and backwards in time.

They progress (on the leader's instructions) to moving *lightly* forwards and backwards while moving the sticks rhythmically. They may have to be told to move on tip-toe to get sufficient lightness into their walk. From this he instructs them to swing the sticks sideways while standing still. Some of the patients manage to move from side to side as well, which adds to the rhythmical effect.

Other variations consist of clapping the sticks together (loudly or softly), and using one stick (held vertically) to tap the floor. Each partner works independently for this. It is possible to extend floor tapping, so that while using the stick to tap the floor the patient moves in a circle round it. This is extremely effective when a large group is working, and the patients get a great deal of pleasure from bringing off a good performance.

A Walk in the Black Forest, relatively short, has to be repeated if all the variations are attempted and sufficient time is given to each one.

6. *Sit and Listen.*—Music: *Waltz* (Act 2, *Faust*), or Chopin's *Nocturne in E flat*. Chairs or stools are arranged in wide circle formation, and the staff and patients sit down to listen to the music. This session not only introduces the patients to good music, but helps to bring about control and discipline in a natural way. See p. 224.

7. *Ball practice*: (*a*) *pat bouncing on the spot, and while moving*; (*b*) *passing between partners*; (*c*) *tossing up and catching.*—

Pat bouncing.—Each patient is given a ball (football, $4\frac{1}{2}$ in. plastic ball or sorbo-rubber ball) and allowed a short session of free practice. The leader suggests a change of activity from time to time. The instructors move around, coaching and generally assisting the patients.

a. On the spot.—The patient keeps the ball bouncing by patting it on the ground with the palm of the hand. He should use one hand at first; later, each hand in turn. Variations: high, medium, and low bouncing.

Progressions consist of pat bouncing while moving freely about the hall, using one hand only, and avoiding other 'bouncers'. Later, each hand should be used in turn.

This is followed by pat bouncing into a circle. A small circle is drawn on the floor. The patients, two or three to a circle, move around pat bouncing a ball into the circle. They must take it in turn to pat the ball. If the ball fails to enter the circle the players must stop and start again. The smaller the circle the more difficult the practice becomes.

b. Passing between partners.—Partners stand opposite each other, the distance varying according to ability. (*a*) They throw the ball to and fro without allowing it to drop. (*b*) The same, but partners change position. Thus A throws to B, and they quickly change position before B returns the ball to A. (*c*) The ball is bounced from partner to partner, the distance between being gradually increased. (*d*) Throw and bounce alternately from one to the other. The ball is first passed in the air and then bounced on the floor. This is useful for teaching timing.

c. Tossing up and catching.—Each patient has a ball. (*a*) He throws it up into the air and catches it as many times as possible while standing still. (*b*) The same, but he moves freely about the hall. (*c*) He throws the ball up into the air and allows it to bounce on the floor before catching it. (*d*) He throws the ball high into the air and claps his hands a given number of times before catching it. (*e*) As before, but moving freely about the hall. (*f*) Throwing the ball up high into the air and turning about before catching it; clapping can be added to this.

8. *Mime: Ghosts and watchers.*—Music: Sibelius's *Valse Triste.* Generally a very popular activity. This is surprising, in a way, because it is usually necessary to explain what a ghost (and a watcher) is. It helps to give a demonstration of a ghost with the aid of a sheet.

A number of patients are chosen as watchers; they are supposed to be keen on ghost spotting, and are sitting at midnight in the old kitchen of a haunted farmhouse deep in the heart of the country. (Obviously there is plenty of room for imagination here.)

The rest of the patients are various types of ghosts: tall, thin ghosts who make thin wailing noises; ghosts with fluttering hands; ghosts who are tall and silent and stealthy; ghosts who clump their way along, heavy-footed and ponderous.

The watchers sit on stools or chairs in a circle at the end of the hall. The ghosts are formed up in file, one behind the other, at the opposite end. The watchers look around them, showing anxiety, apprehension, fear, and alarm as they 'sense' the presence of the phantoms. The ghosts, strictly in character, advance slowly in line towards the watchers, becoming increasingly menacing as they draw near.

They circle the watchers, acting in a terrifying manner. On the second circling some of the ghosts (who have previously marked down victims) approach them closely. The watchers involved immediately drop dead, and fall off their chairs or stools on to the floor. It is wise to have mats or mattresses around the watchers' area.

The ghosts circle again; this time some of them touch the 'dead' watchers, who immediately come to life and join the ghosts. They can link up with a partner or move in file.

Throughout the mime the leader constantly adjusts the volume of the music, raising and lowering it to heighten the drama. As each of the watchers falls dead the tambour can be struck strongly to increase the dramatic effect.

9. *Activity with a hoop*—'*Anything you like ...*'—Music: Ravel's *Bolero*. Each patient is given a hoop, 24 in. or 30 in. in diameter. The group listen to a short extract from the *Bolero*, and the leader emphasizes the underlying rhythm.

The patients are then encouraged to move out into the main body of the hall, so that there is plenty of space around them, and try out any movements they like to the music. It is pointed out that the movements must be of their own invention, not exercises they have been taught, and that they can do them while walking or standing still.

A few produce good individual movement patterns; others have little idea of what they are aiming at and either copy or perform set exercises.

It is important not to let this period go on for too long. Three or four minutes is sufficient.

10. *Percussion band. Variations*: (*a*) *group playing*; (*b*) *section playing*; (*c*) *standing and sitting*; (*d*) *walking round the circle*.— Music: *Spanish Flea*. This is a progression on the percussion activity described on p. 221. As before, the patients sit in a wide

circle on stools or chairs facing inward. Two of the instructors stand inside the circle.

The instructors give out the instruments, remembering the likes and dislikes of the patients (p. 222). Meanwhile the leader spins his record and asks the patients to listen to the music and get the rhythm.

When the gong sounds the patients tackle their instruments with enthusiasm. First they work as a group, with the instructors and the leader helping them to keep time. The leader then suggests that various sections of the group should work with certain instruments only: thus one section is limited to triangles, another to Indian bells, a third to clappers, and so on. He then 'conducts' again, getting first one section to play while the others remain quiet, and then another. So keen are the patients to go on playing that it is generally necessary for him to put a hand out to hush the playing section into silence before pointing his beater at the next section of players. When all sections have had a turn at playing he conducts the group as a whole.

Another variation consists of encouraging the group to change from sitting to standing, plus turning around, while playing. From this they progress to (a) walking in file around the chairs while playing, and (b) walking in and out of the chairs in file.

3. ACTIVITIES FOR THE MILDLY
(AND BORDERLINE) RETARDED

The mildly retarded find music and movement too limited; they need something more purposeful and dynamic. They are capable of tackling a programme made up of informal activities, skipping, relay games, and minor team games, as outlined here. Men and women take part in the same programme.

The borderline handicapped need an ordinary well-balanced programme of games and gymnastics. This type of approach is essential for young, physically fit psychopaths. Swimming fits well into the programme. It is important to divide the men and women into separate groups.

Suitable games for men include five-a-side football, volley-ball, table-tennis, soccer, and cricket. For women netball, volley-ball, table-tennis, and badminton are particularly useful.

Aims of treatment.—See p. 208.

Programme sequence for mildly retarded.—Alternative programmes are used to provide variety. One is made up of activities and games, with some music; the other consists of 'potted sports'.

In arranging the first type of programme it is important to start with an activity which gets the group moving as a whole. The middle section should have a quiet period, e.g., Sit and listen or a suitable mime. The final item consists of a team game.

The organization of a potted sports session is described on p. 243.

SPECIMEN PROGRAMME: ACTIVITIES AND GAMES
(For ambulant patients)

1. Activity: Four walls change.
2. Skipping: (*a*) individual, on the spot and travelling; (*b*) group work. *Stars and Stripes Forever*, *Liberty Bell*, etc. (*Sousa the Great*: Columbia TWO 113).
3. Ball practice: (*a*) throwing and catching; (*b*) throwing and changing balls; (*c*) pat bouncing and changing.
4. Mirror movements. Ravel's *Pavane for a Dead Infanta* (Decca SXL 2312).
5. Sit and listen. Chopin's *Waltz in C sharp minor* (Columbia TWO 276).
6. Activity: Circle stick change.
7. Relay game: Circle gap passing.
8. Group game: Tower ball.
9. Minor team game: Circle hand ball.

SPECIMEN PROGRAMME: POTTED SPORTS
(For ambulant patients)

1. Goal shooting: netball or basket-ball goal.
2. Quoits: large wooden quoit board with long pegs (wall mounted).
3. Skittles: 12 arranged in arrow-head formation.
4. Wall-ball: padder-bat and 'gamster' plastic ball.

DESCRIPTION OF ACTIVITIES AND GAMES

1. *Activity: Four walls change.*—The group is divided up into four teams, all the players wearing coloured bands.

Each team is lined up against a wall. At a signal from the leader the players attempt to cross the hall to the opposite wall as quickly as possible.

There is often considerable confusion in the centre, with all the comings and goings. The activity is repeated when the teams have reached their 'new' walls.

A variation consists of starting the activity with the teams facing the walls.

2. *Skipping*: (*a*) *individual, on the spot and travelling*; (*b*) *group work*.—Music: *Stars and Stripes Forever, Liberty Bell*, etc.

a. On the spot.—Each patient is given a ball-bearing rope and told to find a free space in the hall. In *rope swinging forward* the rope is swung from the back, over the head, and under the feet. If performed in 'common time' two springs are taken to one turn of the rope (i.e., skip jump with a rebound). If taken in quick time one spring is made to each turn of the rope. In *rope swinging backward* the rope is swung from the front, over the head, and under the feet from behind. In *high skipping* the performer springs from one foot to the other while raising the knee to about the level of the hip.

Travelling.—All these varieties of skipping can be done while 'travelling': that is, moving forward or backward or sideways. The instructors, who act as coaches, can call out the directions, e.g., "Move forwards! Now backwards. . . . Move to the right. . . . To the left!"

b. Group skipping.—A rope of about 6–8 yards in length is used. This type of skipping is greatly enjoyed by the patients after the initial difficulty of timing the swinging of the rope has been mastered. Practice should be given in running through and then in entering and leaving from either side. Once proficient many different types of skipping may be tried, e.g., all in before the 4th turn of the rope, skip 12 while in together; all out in 3 turns of the rope.

In all forms of skipping a light easy spring with a good poise of the body should be stressed.

3. *Ball practice*: (*a*) *throwing and catching*; (*b*) *throwing and changing balls*; (*c*) *pat bouncing and changing*.—

a. Throwing and catching.—The patients move freely about the hall, walking or running, throwing a ball up with one hand and catching it with the other, or throwing it up and catching it with the same hand.

b. Throwing and changing.—The patients work in partner formation. Each player has a ball: both players throw at the same time, the balls crossing in the air. Clapping, turning, and the use of right and left hands can be introduced.

c. Pat bouncing and changing.—As previous activity, but the balls are changed by a pat bouncing technique. To keep two balls moving at the same time requires considerable concentration and skill.

4. *Mirror movements.*—Music: Ravel's *Pavane for a Dead Infanta.* This is a useful and very pleasant activity. The group is arranged in pairs; they are told to space themselves out over the hall, so that each pair has plenty of room to move.

Partners face each other, standing close together. One has to imitate the actions of the other, as if looking into a mirror. At first the movements are confined to the arms, and one arm only is used at a time. It is important that the performers do not touch each other. When carrying out the arm movements the palms of the hands should be facing, but held about an inch apart. This distance must be maintained during the mirror movements.

The arm actions can consist of any simple rhythmical movements: circlings, movements sideways, upwards, or downwards.

Having practised individual arm movements successfully with the music (and each arm should be used in turn) the leader suggests that each performer should drift away some distance from his partner before returning to link up with him again. Another progression consists of both performers turning sideways on, with one hand almost in contact, and then walking round the hall to the music. They then resume their facing positions and continue their mirror dancing. A further progression consists of each performer leaving his partner and finding another. The performers walk anywhere in the hall, meet, link up, and perform their mirror movements.

When individual arm movements can be carried out successfully, the performers use both arms: the movements then become much more interesting. It should be noted that whatever form of arm movement is carried out the performers should always allow generalized movement of the body to occur, so that there is nothing stilted or restrained about the activity.

5. *Sit and listen.*—Music: Chopin's *Waltz in C sharp minor.* Chairs or stools are arranged in wide circle formation, and the staff and patients sit down and listen to the music. *See* p. 224.

6. *Activity: Circle stick change.*—The group is divided into two or three teams. Each team forms a circle, the players being well spaced. Each player has a stick (broomstick or ash stick) which he

holds in the upright position in one hand, with the end resting on the floor. The stick is held at arm's length from the body.

On the signal 'Change!' from the instructor in charge of each team, the players move up one place (in either a clockwise or anticlockwise direction, as previously arranged), letting go of their sticks and attempting to grasp the adjoining ones, so as to prevent them falling. The process is repeated, each team trying to have the least number of casualties among its sticks.

When the players can move up one place at a time without letting the sticks fall, they attempt a move of two places.

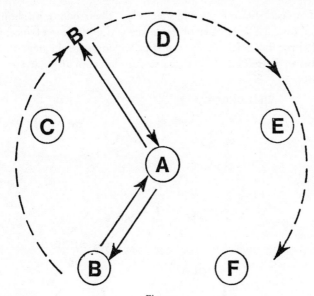

Fig. 202.

7. *Relay game*: *Circle gap passing.*—The group is divided into three or four teams of six or more players. Each team is arranged in circle formation, with one player (A) in the centre with a football. There should be plenty of space between the circle players, and it should be the same for each team. To ensure accuracy the players' positions should be marked out on the floor; the central point of the circle should also be marked out.

Player A (in the centre) throws the ball to player B, who returns it and immediately runs behind player C to the next gap (*Fig.* 202).

Here he receives the ball again from A, and returns it to him, running behind D to the next gap, and so on, until he returns to his original place. During this players C, D, E, and F remain stationary.

Player A then passes the ball to player C, who runs round in the same way as previously described, receiving and returning the ball in each gap. Players D, E, and F also run round the circle in the same way when it is their turn.

The first team to complete the course properly and get the ball back to their central player is the winner.

8. *Group game: Tower ball.*—The players, who have two footballs between them, form a large circle. Their positions should be marked out. In the centre of the circle is the tower—a tripod made up of three ash sticks or broomsticks, tied securely near the top. The tower is defended by three or four players (*Fig.* 203).

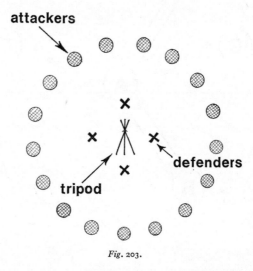

Fig. 203.

The object of the game is for the attackers to throw in the balls and knock down the tower.

The leader gives the signal to begin. The defenders use their arms and legs to stop the ball and shield the tower, but are not allowed to kick. When the attackers succeed in knocking down the tower they run to a wall or line. The defenders run after them and try and tag them. The tagged players now become defenders.

Should the defenders knock the tower down they must erect it as quickly as possible. No attacker may step inside the circle.

The game needs to be coached well: the attackers should not be allowed to put too much force into their throwing.

9. *Minor team game*: *Circle hand ball.*—The group is divided into two or three teams. Each team forms a circle, the players standing with their legs astride. Each team has two or three footballs, and is coached by an instructor.

At a signal from their instructor the players with footballs attempt to pass them through other players' legs by batting them along the floor with the hand. The 'attacked' players try and prevent this by bringing their legs together, jumping up, or twisting the body around. If the ball passes through a player's legs he leaves the game. Once the game is started all the players have a chance of getting a ball.

The team with the most players (when the stop signal is given) wins.

A variation can be played in sitting, stools or chairs being arranged in circle formation. Instead of batting the ball with the hand each player has a broomstick and pokes it along.

ORGANIZING POTTED SPORTS

Much of the success of a potted sports session depends on good organization. The equipment required must be laid out in the recreation hall before the patients are due in—the corners acting as areas for the four events—and the staff taking part must know exactly what they are expected to do. Any marking out must be done beforehand.

The leader acts as organizer and compère, and is responsible for checking the team scores. If possible, each corner should have its own instructor, who supervises the teams as they compete in his sport.

Teams.—The players are divided into four teams and given coloured identification bands. Each team appoints a captain, who is responsible for the behaviour of his players. He decides the order in which they play, and may also be able to keep the score.

Demonstration.—Each team is allocated to its first sport, and asked to go over to the appropriate corner and sit down on the floor. This avoids any possible confusion. A brief demonstration is then given of the four sports, with clear instructions as to the team procedure to be followed. If each corner is controlled by an instructor he gives his own demonstration and explanation.

Procedure.—The sports start at a whistle signal from the leader. When a team finishes its set of activities the players sit on the floor and wait until all the teams have finished play. The captain checks his score with the instructor.

On a signal from the leader all the teams change corners. Prior to this he has clearly indicated the new areas for each team. This procedure is followed until all the teams have participated in the four sports.

METHOD OF PLAY

Corner 1. *Goal-shooting: netball or basket-ball goal.*—Players in file. A cross on the floor indicates the 'shooting' base. To maintain interest each player shoots once and then goes to the back of the file. The score is recorded. The file rotates three to six times.

Corner 2. *Quoits: large wooden quoit board with long pegs (wall mounted).*—Players in file. A cross on the floor indicates the throwing base. Each player is allowed three quoits. He throws them—the score is taken—and he goes to the back of the file. The file rotates three to six times.

Corner 3. *Skittles:* 12 *arranged in arrow-head formation.*—Players in file. A cross on the floor indicates the bowling base. Each player is allowed three balls. He plays them—the score is taken—and he goes to the back of the file. *No* rotation of file because of time required in retrieving and setting up skittles.

Corner 4. *Wall-ball: padder-bat and 'gamster' plastic ball.*—Each player in turn bats the ball against the wall while standing on a marked line (about 9 ft. from wall). The aim is to maintain a continuous flow of 25 hits. A large circle drawn, or pinned, on the wall indicates the target area.

CHAPTER XXVI

MUSIC AND MOVEMENT
IN THE TREATMENT OF THE MENTALLY ILL

MUSIC and movement forms a valuable part of the recreational therapy programme used in psychiatric hospitals. Combined with well-chosen mime and game-form activities, and handled by instructors with personality and leadership ability, it is capable of a wide application in the treatment of both men and women patients.

Whenever possible, music and movement should be carried out in a recreation hall or gymnasium. Improvised sessions can be organized in ward day-rooms, but the range of activities is considerably limited.

SELECTION OF PATIENTS

Three main groups of patients benefit from music and movement:—

1. Ambulant long-stay patients, mainly chronic schizophrenics. This group includes those who have retained most of their personality characteristics, and those with deteriorating behaviour and fragmented personalities. The latter may require a secure environment.

2. Ambulant and non-ambulant psycho-geriatric patients. Many are confused and demented.

3. Acute patients, mainly in the younger age-group, who suffer from a wide range of psychiatric illnesses. These include the functional psychoses (schizophrenia, endogenous depression, manic depressive psychoses); the neuroses (anxiety states, hysteria, reactive depression, obsessional and phobic states); psychopathic personality; and personality disorders (inadequacy and immaturity).

The patients will be treated either in the acute admission wards or the day hospital.

LONG-STAY PATIENTS
(MAINLY CHRONIC SCHIZOPHRENICS)

These patients, mostly middle-aged or elderly, are not only asocial and withdrawn, but often completely institutionalized. Few are likely to be discharged. They have little drive or initiative and, if left to their own devices, sit around doing nothing. They withdraw into their own world of fantasy.

Chronic schizophrenics suffer from psychomotor retardation, characterized by slowness of initiative and slowness of execution: they are incapable of moving in a spontaneous free manner, as is normal, and their movements appear limited and restricted. Their sense of position and body-awareness is also considerably lessened.

Many of these patients require maintenance doses of tranquillizing drugs, such as Largactil. It is important that the drugs are regularly reviewed by their consultants.

PLANNED ACTIVITY

Some chronic schizophrenics are capable of simple repetitive work, and attend the industrial therapy department. Usually they are employed on routine jobs, such as folding or stamping paper bags used for sterile supplies.

Some of the patients, however, are not capable of this. They need a regular daily programme of recreational activities to break up their monotony and prevent them from becoming totally inactive. Suitable activities include simple games (the childhood ones are often best, e.g., rounders), listening to music, going for walks and outings, and taking part in music and movement classes.

Aims of treatment.—The patients must be kept fully ambulant and mobile. An attempt must also be made to make them aware of what is going on around them. This includes endeavouring to arouse their interest in their dress, personal hygiene, and social behaviour. Many are completely indifferent to the way in which they dress or how they look. Men will walk around in public with their trouser flies gaping open, women with their knickers half-down.

Problems of communicating.—The difficulty of communicating and 'getting through' to chronic schizophrenics is formidable, to say the least. Recreational therapists must be prepared to use great patience. They must bear in mind the fact that any improvement in a patient's attitude or behaviour pattern can only be expected over a long period of time: months or years.

It is important that continuity of staff is maintained whenever possible. Frequent changes of staff tend to disturb these patients, and may well lead to a negative response. When a change is necessary at least one member of the original staff should be left.

A high staff–patient ratio is important. When exercise therapy is first attempted this may necessitate one instructor per patient. Later on group training is possible, provided only a small number of patients is allocated to each group.

MUSIC AND MOVEMENT

Only a few very simple activities are attempted at the beginning. For example, the instructor attempts to persuade a patient to shake a percussion instrument to music of a strong rhythmical nature (p. 222), or catch a ball when it is thrown to him. At first the patient may hold the instrument but fail to shake it; similarly, he may let the ball either strike him or pass by without evincing the slightest interest.

When the patient makes a positive response the instructor must show appreciation and give a 'booster' dose of praise. This encourages him to do the right thing again.

Walking to music.—Walking in circle formation to background music—small individual groups of patients being involved with their instructors—is very useful. The patients walk in file or sideways with linked arms or hands. Progression is achieved by creating several smaller circles; this produces a more individual participation.

The music should be bright and stimulating, e.g., Jankowski's *A Walk in the Black Forest*, Eric Coates's *The Merrymakers Overture*, and Sousa's *Stars and Stripes Forever*.

When circular walking is established 'stopping' to command— a note on the tambour, for example—is introduced. Rhythmical clapping can also be added to the walking.

Another useful activity consists of organizing small groups of patients into circle formation and then instructing them to wander anywhere they like. The therapist adds: "Each person you meet . . . touch his hand. Touch two hands . . .." Later, he says: "Nod to each other when you meet. Nod and shake hands . . .."

Simple mimes.—Very simple mimes may be tried, such as 'painting' an imaginary picture or 'strolling' down a street. For 'painting' the instructor helps with the 'collection' of canvas, rags, easel, and brushes. Large outsize strokes are made in painting the canvas, the 'artist' moving back from time to time to inspect his work. In 'strolling' the patients walk down a 'street', looking into shop windows and avoiding the traffic. They greet other strollers, shaking hands and chatting.

Music is used for both mimes. *The Largo* from Dvořák's *New World* Symphony seems to inspire the 'painters', and Vaughan Williams's *Seventeen Come Sunday* keeps the strollers moving nicely.

LONG-STAY PATIENTS
(MAINLY CHRONIC SCHIZOPHRENICS)
WHO MAY REQUIRE A SECURE ENVIRONMENT

These are middle-aged patients with fragmented personalities and deteriorating behaviour. Few are likely to be discharged from hospital. They need a regular programme of simple physical activities which will not only provide them with some all-round exercise, but give them enjoyment and a change of environment.

Music and movement is an excellent way of achieving this. (*See* specimen programmes, pp. 220–237.) It has the advantage, too, of being comparatively easy to organize in a secure environment.

AMBULANT PSYCHO-GERIATRIC PATIENTS

These patients, whose ages range from 65 to 90 years, are often confused and demented. Some are blind or deaf. A number, too, are disabled to a varying degree by arthritis or paralysis (usually the result of a 'stroke'). Some suffer from diabetes. Many are incontinent, despite intensive toilet training. Incontinence is particularly likely to occur as the patients deteriorate.

The majority, because of their confused state, cannot concentrate; as a result they may sit about all day doing nothing, or wander, sometimes in a severe state of agitation. The periods of confusion, however, alternate with transient lucid intervals. In these intervals the patients are capable of holding a normal conversation.

In time the patients become more and more child-like in their responses. Indeed, as their memory deteriorates, childhood matters are the only ones well remembered.

Communication.—These patients are extremely difficult to get 'through' to, although in their moments of lucidity it is possible to communicate in a normal way. A little later, however, they may be hopelessly confused and demented.

Aims of treatment.—The patients must be kept fully mobile and ambulant. An attempt must be made to stimulate and arouse their interest in their own care and in outside matters. In choosing activities it is essential to remember the patients' age, and their general degree of frailty, and to avoid anything which is too strenuous or demanding.

Graduated activity is not only important from the point of view of maintaining function, but of helping to maintain the normal waking–sleeping pattern. This is essential if the patients are to sleep properly at night.

Recreational Therapy Programme

A regular daily programme of recreational activities must be arranged. It consists of games (from draughts and ludo to 'snap'), listening to lively music, and taking part in simple sessions of music and movement. Medleys of old-time songs are ideal for 'listening' periods; the patients join in and let themselves go.

Music and movement.—Most of the activities are carried out in sitting. They can be based on those described in the programme given on p. 220, which includes a percussion band and game-form activities with balls, hoops, beanbags, and quoits. Because of the patients' age, however, a number of items must be modified or deleted, e.g., marching musical chairs.

Staff–patient ratio.—Psycho-geriatric patients need patience and an unhurried relaxed approach. A fairly high staff–patient ratio, 1 : 5 for example, is required if the music and movement sessions are to be successfully carried out.

NON-AMBULANT PSYCHO-GERIATRIC PATIENTS

Many of these patients are senile with advanced dementia. Nearly all suffer from the associated illnesses and disabilities of old age: diabetes, arthritis, and hemiplegia. Incontinence, because of deterioration and inactivity, is commonplace.

The majority of the patients need feeding and shaving. Help with dressing is also necessary.

Recreational therapy.—A regular programme of the type described for ambulant patients in the previous section is essential. Many of the music and movement activities will have to be scaled down to their simplest form, however. A high staff–patient ratio is essential, e.g., 1 : 5.

Aims of treatment.—The patients must be kept mobile and out of bed for as long as possible; that is, until the final phase of deterioration sets in. An attempt must be made to stimulate their interest in outside things.

Specific therapy.—Specific exercises, passive movements, and walking re-education will be needed for a number of patients, to prevent contractures and maintain function. This applies particularly to the hemiplegics and arthritics. In some cases treatment must be reinforced by simple forms of heat therapy, e.g., wax baths and infra-red radiation.

ACUTE PATIENTS

1. Patients Treated in the Acute Admission Wards or the Day Hospital

These patients, mainly in the younger age-group, suffer from a wide range of psychiatric illnesses. They include the functional psychoses, the neuroses, psychopathic personality, and personality disorders. (*See* p. 245.)

Where the admission wards of the main hospital have the necessary facilities the full range of treatment, including occupational and recreational therapy, will be undertaken. Where space is limited, however, the patients may be sent to the day hospital for their occupational and recreational activities. A programme of activities is outlined on p. 237.

2. Patients with Behaviour Disorders who Require a Secure Environment

These are young or middle-aged men and women. Some are subject to violent behaviour; some have suicidal tendencies. Others are persistent criminals and persistent absconders. A few are sex offenders; some have psychopathic personalities. They all need to be in secure hospital conditions, not only for their own good but for the safety of society.

Some of the patients require secure conditions over a period of several years. During their stay in hospital considerable help is necessary in building up long-term habits of accepted behaviour and work, and stable relationships with others.

Treatment.—The patients need industrial therapy and a wide range of educational and social facilities. They must be able to attend evening classes, soccer matches and the cinema, and participate in organized outings. The need for security should not limit the scope of the therapeutic programme. Patients attend outside activities either individually or in very small groups, accompanied by members of the nursing staff.

Physical education.—A regular well-organized programme of physical activities is required. Whenever possible men and women take part in the same exercise sessions. Some of the more strenuous activities, such as agility work and soccer, must be limited to men.

The programme should include swimming, informal physical education, and games. Major games, such as soccer, basket-ball, and volley-ball, are particularly important. Special interests should be included, such as weight-training or athletics.

THE DAY HOSPITAL

Most large psychiatric hospitals have associated day hospitals or centres with accommodation for some sixty to a hundred patients. Patients living at home attend on a day basis from Monday to Friday. Some centres provide combined facilities for day and in-patients.

1. ACUTE PATIENTS

In centres taking both day and in-patients the range of psychiatric conditions treated is very wide (p. 245). In general, the majority of patients are in the younger age group; the average age is about 40.

Treatment.—Treatment is by chemotherapy, individual and group psychotherapy, and physical methods, such as electro-convulsion therapy. It is supplemented by a programme of occupational and recreational activities, as outlined below on p. 252.

2. Chronic Patients

Other day centres are chiefly concerned with giving support to chronic patients.

Aims of treatment.—There are three main aims:—

1. To give support to the chronic patient by (*a*) suitable psychotherapy and chemotherapy, and (*b*) participation in a programme of recreational and occupational activities which expand his interests.

2. To give reassurance and encouragement of the right sort. This applies not only to the patient's efforts to participate in his programme of physical activities, but to his attempt to lead a normal life outside. It is important that the patients must want to attend the centre and take part in the activities prescribed.

3. To assist the patient to continue in a normal work pattern during periods of unemployment as, for example, when he loses his job. He then attends the industrial therapy unit until he is fixed up with another job.

Treatment for Acute and Chronic Patients

Occupational and recreational programme.—A wide range of activities is used: art, musical appreciation, drama, housecraft, woodwork, discussion groups, physical education, games, and all types of dancing.

In addition, outside visits are arranged to the theatre, the seaside and local events, such as flower-shows and athletic meetings.

Informal physical education.—A useful programme consists of an introductory period of warming up activities to music (in sitting and standing), followed by a short session of relaxation exercises in sitting, and a games period: relay and minor team games. The programme ends with a major game, e.g., volley-ball. Usually, both men and women patients attend the same session.

Games are particularly helpful in bringing about better social behaviour. They not only cultivate the team spirit but a desire to do the right or 'accepted' thing.

APPENDIX

EXERCISE TERMINOLOGY

THROUGHOUT this book the terminology used to describe the exercises is based on the *Terminology of Swedish Educational Gymnastics*. Some of the exercises described have starting

ADDITIONAL DERIVED POSITIONS

POSITION	ABBREVIATION	EXPLANATION
	a. Of Arms from Standing	
Forearm reach standing	Forearm rch. st.	The elbows are flexed to 90°, with the palms facing each other. (*See Fig.* 127, p. 102.)
Drag standing	drag st.	The arms are raised backward as far as possible, with the palms facing inward. (*See Fig.* 56 A, p. 49.)
	b. Of Trunk from Lying	
Fixed high thigh support across prone lying	fix. high thigh sup. acr. pr. ly.	As prone lying, but the thighs rest across apparatus, such as two balance benches, placed one on top of the other. The trunk, head, and legs form a straight line. (*See Fig.* 38, p. 41.)

OBLIQUE STRETCH POSITIONS OF ARMS: SIMPLIFIED TERMINOLOGY

STANDARD TERMINOLOGY	SUGGESTED TERMINOLOGY	EXPLANATION OF POSITION
Oblique downward forward stretch standing	Low reach standing	The arms are held midway between reach position and the normal position by the sides of the body. (*See Fig.* 157, p. 132, which shows the low reach grasp position.)
Oblique upward forward stretch standing	High reach standing	As reach position, but the arms are held midway between reach and stretch positions. (*See Fig.* 113, p. 89.)
Oblique downward sideways stretch standing	Low yard standing	The arms are held midway between the yard position and the normal position by the sides of the body.
Oblique upward sideways stretch standing	High yard standing	The arms are held midway between yard and stretch positions.

positions which are not included in this terminology. In describing exercises in which the oblique stretch positions are assumed, a simplified terminology has been used. For additions and modifications *see* previous page.

GYMNASTIC TERMS: USE OF 'SINGLE' AND 'ALTERNATE'

The terms *single* and *alternate* are often confused; they are defined here.

SINGLE.—The term is used when one arm (or leg) is moved *in turn* with the other arm (or leg), or when one arm (or leg) is moved *several times* in succession before the other arm (or leg) is exercised, e.g., (*a*) Standing; single Arm raising forward, (*b*) Forearm reach sitting; single Forearm turning inward and outward continuously to a given count.

Single is also used when one limb only is to be exercised; the term is then qualified by additional information, e.g., Reach grasp high half standing (beam and block); single (affected) Leg swinging forward and backward.

ALTERNATE.—The term is used when one arm (or leg) moves towards one limit of the movement while the other arm (or leg) moves towards the other limit, e.g., Walk forward standing; alternate Arm swinging forward and backward.

REFERENCE

Terminology of Swedish Educational Gymnastics. Physical Education Association of Great Britain and Northern Ireland (formerly Ling Physical Education Association): 1950. London.

BIBLIOGRAPHY

GENERAL SURGERY

AIRD, I. (1957), *A Companion in Surgical Studies*, 2nd ed. Edinburgh: E. & S. Livingstone.

BEESLY, L., and JOHNSON, T. B. (1939), *Manual of Surgical Anatomy*, 5th ed. London : Oxford University Press.

MILES, A., and LEARMONTH, J. (1950), *Operative Surgery*, 3rd ed. London: Oxford University Press.

PHYSICAL EDUCATION

BUKH, N. (1939), *Primary Gymnastics*, 5th ed. London: Methuen.

CHRISTENSEN, L. E., and TRAP, P. M. (1938), *Textbook of Gymnastics*, 1st ed. London: University of London Press.

KNUDSEN, K. A. (1947), *Textbook of Gymnastics*, 2nd ed. London: J. & A. Churchill.

Ling Physical Education Association (1950), *Terminology of Swedish Educational Gymnastics*. London.

MORGAN, R. E., and ADAMSON, G. T. (1961), *Circuit Training*, 2nd ed. London : G. Bell & Sons.

MUNROW, A. D. (1963), *Pure and Applied Gymnastics*, 2nd ed. London: Edward Arnold.

THULIN, J. G. (1947), *Gymnastic Handbook*, 1st ed. Lund: South Swedish Gymnastic Institute.

ORTHOPÆDIC SURGERY

SMILLIE, I. S. (1962), *Injuries of the Knee Joint*, 3rd ed. Edinburgh: E. & S. Livingstone.

WATSON-JONES, R. (1955), *Fractures and Joint Injuries*, 4th ed. Edinburgh: E. & S. Livingstone.

WILES, P., and SWEETNAM, R. (1965), *Essentials of Orthopædics*, 4th ed. London: J. & A. Churchill.

PHYSICAL TREATMENT

CASH, J. E. (1950), *Textbook of Medical Conditions for Physiotherapists*, 1st ed. London: Faber and Faber.

GARDINER, M. D. (1953), *Principles of Exercise Therapy*, 1st ed. London: G. Bell & Sons.

MENNELL, J. (1940), *Physical Treatment*, 4th ed. London: J. & A. Churchill.

TIDY, N. M. (1968), *Massage and Remedial Exercises*, 11th ed. Bristol: John Wright.

MENTAL ILLNESS

CURRAN, D., and PARTRIDGE, M. (1972), *Psychological Medicine: An Introduction to Psychiatry*, 6th ed. Edinburgh: E. & S. Livingstone.

HENDERSON, D. K., and GILLESPIE, R. D. (1969), *A Textbook of Psychiatry*, 10th ed. London: Oxford University Press.

MENTAL RETARDATION

HEATON-WARD, W. A. (1975), *Mental Subnormality*, 4th ed. Bristol: John Wright.

KIRMAN, B. H. (1968), *Mental Retardation*, 1st ed. London: Pergamon.

MORRIS, PAULINE (1969), *Put Away*, 1st ed. London: Routledge & Kegan Paul.

TREGOLD, R. F., and SODDY, K. (1970), *Mental Retardation*, 11th ed. London: Baillière, Tindall and Cassell.

INDEX